THE HEALTHY INSTANT POT COOKBOOK

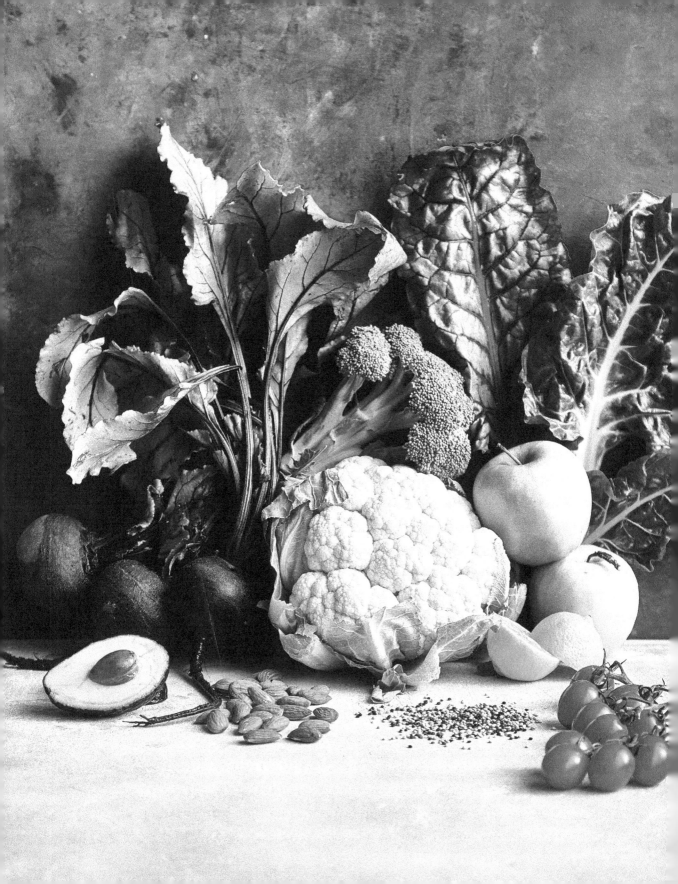

KAREN LEE YOUNG

the healthy instant pot
COOKBOOK

 75

LOW-CALORIE RECIPES MADE EASY

ROCKRIDGE
PRESS

For general information on our other products and services or to obtain technical support, please contact our Customer Care Department within the United States at (866) 744-2665, or outside the United States at (510) 253-0500.

Rockridge Press publishes its books in a variety of electronic and print formats. Some content that appears in print may not be available in electronic books, and vice versa.

TRADEMARKS: Rockridge Press and the Rockridge Press logo are trademarks or registered trademarks of Callisto Media Inc. and/or its affiliates, in the United States and other countries, and may not be used without written permission. All other trademarks are the property of their respective owners. Rockridge Press is not associated with any product or vendor mentioned in this book.

Interior and Cover Designer: Rachel Haeseker
Art Producer: Sara Feinstein
Editor: Kelly Koester
Production Manager: Martin Worthington

Copyright Page: Photography © 2021 Hélène Dujardin, cover; © Hélène Dujardin, pp. ii, 100; © Elysa Weitala, p. vi; © Marija Vidal, pp.viii, 18, 70, 92, 104; © Nadine Greeff, pp. x, 22, 38, 46, 60, 66, 96, 110, 132; © Andrew Purcell, pp. 26, 62,122; © Darren Muir, pp. 34, 86; © Evi Abeler, pp. 42, 54, 128, 134; Shutterstock, pp. 50, 76; © Thomas J. Story, p. 80; © Becky Stayner, p.114; © Annie Martin, p. 118; Trent Lanz/Stocksy, p. 136; © Kate Sears, p. 138. Food Styling by Anna Hampton, cover.

Paperback ISBN: 978-1-63807-016-0
eBook ISBN: 978-1-63807-515-8

R0

To James and Scarlett, my favorite people to cook for.

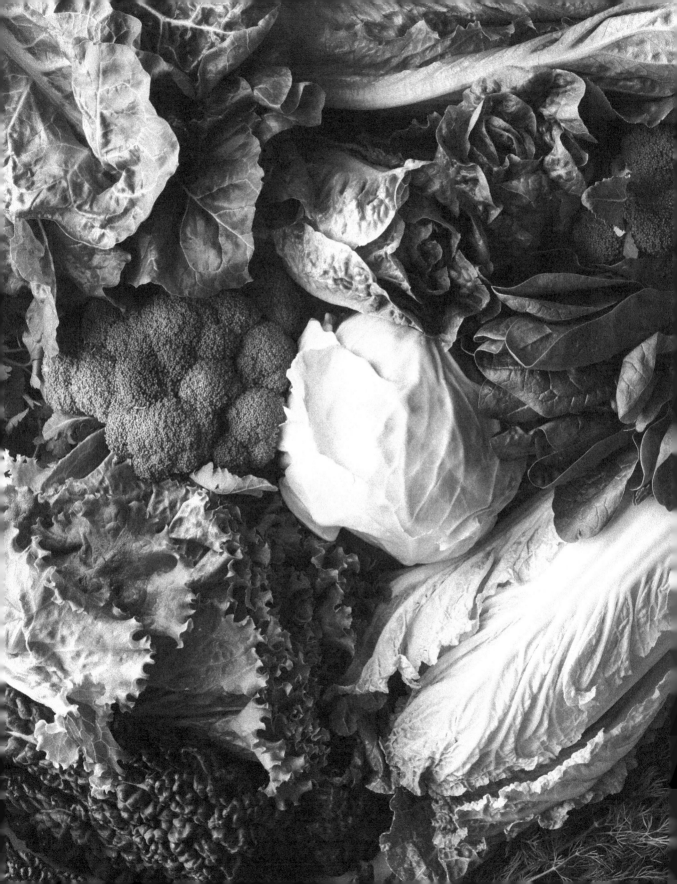

CONTENTS

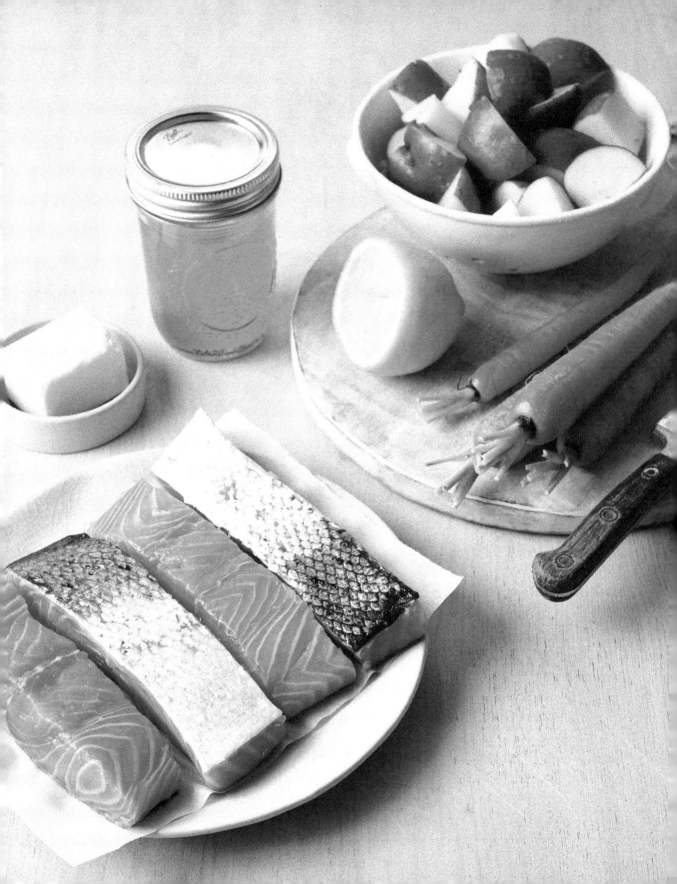

INTRODUCTION

Do you want to eat healthily and create delicious, wholesome meals, yet don't want to spend hours in the kitchen each day? Great! You're in the right place. When it comes to cooking nutritious and well-rounded meals, the Instant Pot is perfect for the job.

The Instant Pot is one of the most popular kitchen appliances for home cooks. I must admit, I resisted using it for as long as I could until I heard about the many benefits of Instant Pot cooking. Dried beans can be cooked without presoaking overnight? Ribs become fall-off-the-bone tender in less than an hour? Stocks and sauces can be made without the need to stir and monitor the stove? I was sold.

Between the hissing sound, the different buttons and settings, and pressure release knob, I was intimidated and terrified the first time I used the Instant Pot. Over time, I became more comfortable with the many features of this versatile kitchen appliance and started experimenting with a wide variety of healthy dishes. Not only is it easy to eat lots of wholesome, unprocessed foods, but also I'm more likely to whip up a last-minute healthy meal instead of resorting to processed foods and takeout.

Eating and cooking healthy food can be a challenge for many, especially if you are cooking for a family. These days in our house—with an energetic toddler who is constantly exploring and running around—cooking needs to be fast, effortless, and with little hands-on time. The Instant Pot quickly became a fixture on our kitchen counter. With the Instant Pot, you can set it, let it work its magic, and come back at mealtime to enjoy a delicious, healthy meal with your family.

One misconception many people have is that healthy food is bland and boring. This isn't the case here. Healthy cooking can be full of flavor and satisfying. With that in mind, I wrote this book to share with you a collection of healthy Instant Pot recipes that are certainly not lacking in flavor. From Southwestern Tofu Scramble (page 68) to Balsamic-Glazed Pork Tenderloin (page 120) and Poached Pears with Cardamom (page 124), I'm sure there's a recipe you'll enjoy.

This book is designed for anyone, whether you're new to electric pressure cooking or just looking for different tastes to add to your rotation. No matter what your health goals or culinary experience may be, I'm confident that this book will help you discover how easy and enjoyable healthy cooking can be. Even if you've never plugged your Instant Pot into the wall before, the recipes in this book will show you how to get the most out of this versatile appliance.

I hope you'll use these recipes as a starting point and come up with your own healthy creations. Let's get cooking!

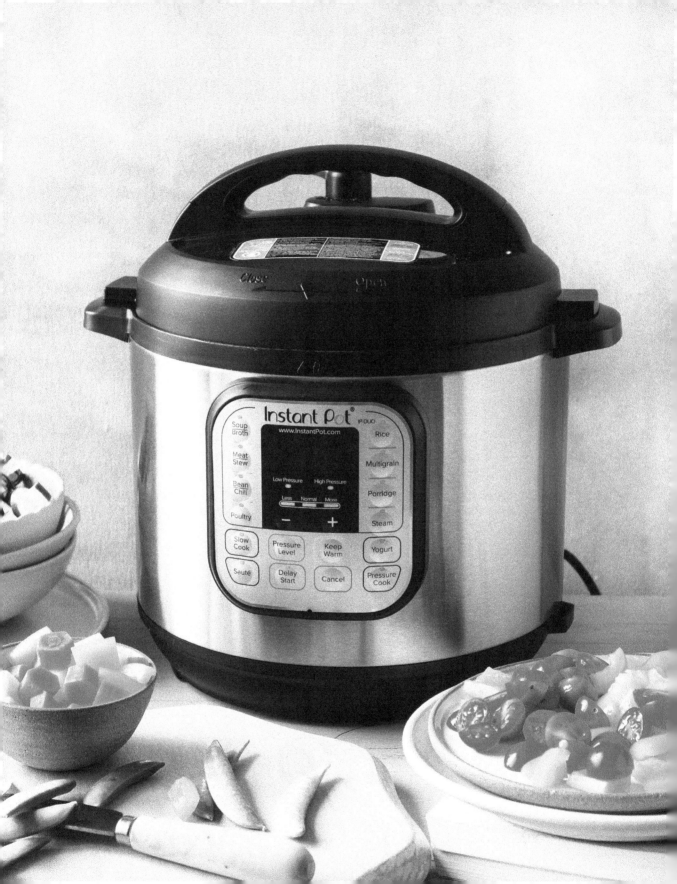

CHAPTER ONE

Healthy Cooking with the Power of the Instant Pot

Cooking healthy meals doesn't have to be complicated. In this chapter, I'll cover the basics of using the Instant Pot to cook healthy meals. I will also highlight some of the kitchen tools that will help you along the way and recommend healthy staples you'll need to get a nutritious and delicious meal on the table with little effort.

The Easiest Way to Cook for Your Health

If you've picked up this book, you are likely looking for some healthy changes for the way you cook and eat. Congratulations on making this positive choice! No matter what your health goals may be—whether you want to lose weight, maintain the same weight, or eat for general health and longevity—the Instant Pot can help you toward your goals.

Here are some reasons why the Instant Pot is so well suited for healthy cooking:

Minimal use of oil or fat: With its wide range of programmable settings, the Instant Pot is an extremely versatile kitchen appliance. The most popular cooking function—pressure cooking—is an excellent way to cook meat, vegetables, and grains to perfection with less oil or other fats than other cooking methods, such as browning, braising, sautéing, or pan-frying.

Saves time: The Instant Pot can help you get a healthy and delicious meal on your table fast. Steam pressure builds up inside the sealed pot to achieve a high level of heat in a short period of time, which allows food to cook quickly. Ingredients that usually take a long time to prepare—such as dried beans, grains, and lean meats—can be cooked in a fraction of the time.

Retains nutrients: Boiling and steaming can cause vitamins and minerals to leach out of food and into the water. Since pressure cooking uses less liquid and the overall cooking time is reduced, it preserves more of the nutrients in food compared to other cooking methods.

Perfect for one-pot meals: The Instant Pot allows you to prepare one-pot dishes by adding all the ingredients to the pot at once, setting it, and forgetting it. Many recipes in this book are labeled one-pot meals, which means everything will get cooked at the same time. And there is no need to prepare a separate side dish later, which makes eating healthy easier and quicker with less work.

Hands-off cooking: The Instant Pot is fully automated, which means once you set the cooking time, there is no need to stir continuously or watch the food as it cooks. There is very little risk of burning food in the Instant Pot, so it is a perfect fit for the busy cook. Even better, your meal will be kept warm until you're ready to eat.

My 5 Favorite Healthy Instant Pot Dishes

I hear this question over and over again: What are the best things to cook in the Instant Pot? You can cook just about anything, but here are some dishes in this book that showcase the Instant Pot's ability to cook healthy foods.

1. **Apple-Cinnamon Oatmeal (page 23):** Steel-cut oats usually take a while to cook on the stovetop, but the Instant Pot can get the job done in just minutes with no need for constant stirring. Make a big batch at the beginning of the week, store it in individual serving containers, then reheat it for a fast and satisfying breakfast all week long.

2. **Deviled Eggs (page 45):** Making hard-boiled eggs in the Instant Pot will give you perfect, easy-to-peel eggs every time. These deviled eggs are a tasty appetizer or a delicious, protein-packed snack.

3. **Mushroom-Barley Risotto (page 59):** This is without a doubt the simplest and easiest way to prepare risotto. You can just close the lid and forget all about it until the cooking cycle is finished. There is no need to keep stirring in front of the hot stove!

4. **Teriyaki Chicken Rice Bowls (page 95):** Rice cooks nicely in the Instant Pot. Combined with protein and veggies, it makes for a hearty, well-rounded weeknight meal. The best part is everything gets cooked in one pot, so cleanup is a breeze.

5. **Applesauce (page 130):** Apples cook quickly in the Instant Pot. This naturally sweetened applesauce is terrific to serve alongside roasted pork chops, to use as an oatmeal topping, or to use in baked goods as a substitute for some fats.

A Healthy Approach to Everyday Cooking

Healthy means different things for different people. My approach to healthy cooking is to create delicious, nourishing dishes that get you excited about mealtime. The recipes in this book reflect how I cook for my family—using fresh, wholesome, minimally processed ingredients. As part of a healthy plate, I like to include high-fiber vegetables, lean protein, whole grains, and healthy fats. You will find you can use healthy ingredients to make flavorful, satisfying meals without excessive salt, sugar, or saturated fat.

Before we get into how to use the Instant Pot, let's look at the types of foods found in the healthy recipes in this book.

VEGETABLES

Most vegetables are low in calories but high in fiber, essential minerals, and vitamins. Starchy vegetables like butternut squash and sweet potato add a creamy texture to dishes, while fresh vegetables like corn, carrots, and fennel provide a natural sweetness. Dark, leafy greens such as kale and spinach pack a big nutritional punch, and sneaking them into your daily diet couldn't be simpler. Vegetables quickly soften in the Instant Pot, so they are one of the easiest and quickest things you can make in this appliance.

LEAN PROTEIN

Eating lean cuts of meat, fish, eggs, and legumes with each meal can regulate appetite and help you feel fuller longer. Eggs are rich in high-quality protein and healthy fats, and you will find plenty of egg-based breakfast dishes in this book to help jump-start your day. The Instant Pot is perfect for tenderizing lean or tough cuts of meats, creating a juicy, fall-apart texture. Dried beans are inexpensive and cook quickly in the Instant Pot, so they are a great vegetarian protein option. Fish is an excellent source of omega-3 fatty acids, and eating fish at least once or twice a week is recommended by the American Heart Association. Keep in mind that seafood can get overcooked and chewy if cooked under high pressure for too long, so many of my recipes will call for these ingredients to be added at the end.

HEALTHY CARBS

Diets that avoid carbs have gained popularity in recent years, but not all carbs are created equal. When you eat the right kind, carbs can actually help you achieve and maintain a healthy weight. Complex carbohydrates, which are high in dietary fiber and low in sugar, help you feel satiated because they take more time for your body to digest and break down for energy. In this book, you will find a variety of nutrient-dense recipes using complex carbs such as barley, oats, lentils, sweet potatoes, and chickpeas.

5 Healthy Eating Tips

Although the recipes in this book will help you maintain a healthy diet, there are some simple steps you can take to stick to your new healthy lifestyle.

1. **Keep healthy snacks on hand:** Snack cravings are inevitable, so make sure that you always have some healthy and delicious treats to reach for when the mood strikes. I like to make a batch of Hummus (page 36) at the start of the week to enjoy with vegetables and whole-wheat crackers for a filling and nutritious snack.

2. **Stay hydrated:** Water rehydrates your body and keeps your digestive system moving. If you don't like the taste of plain water, try making some infused water with fresh citrus, mint, or cucumber to add flavor without the unhealthy additives and calories found in many other flavored drinks.

3. **Everything in moderation:** Healthy eating is all about balance. Every once in a while, allow yourself a treat, whether it is a burger or a chocolate bar. The key is to eat them less often and in smaller amounts while balancing them with healthier foods and more physical activity.

4. **Create weekly menus:** Having meals, or at least ideas for meals, planned for the week can help you stay on track with healthy eating goals. You will be less likely to resort to processed foods or opt for takeout when it's 6 o'clock on Thursday and you're feeling hungry and uninspired.

5. **Batch-cook meals to enjoy throughout the week:** Whether you are prepping one meal or a whole week's worth in advance, batch-cooking saves time and allows you to eat well all week long. It makes breakfast, lunch, dinner, and even snacks a snap on days that are particularly busy.

Instant Pot 101

If you already own an Instant Pot (or maybe more than one), you know how they work and what they can do. If you're new to the Instant Pot world, here's a quick rundown of their features and capabilities.

The Instant Pot is an electric multicooker, which means it has several cooking programs. It can function as a pressure cooker (the most popular function), rice cooker, slow cooker, and yogurt-maker. There are preprogrammed settings for various foods, or you can customize the cooking process with the Pressure Cook setting (or Manual, if you own an older model). Either way, the Instant Pot is a game changer for home cooks.

Here are just a few of its advantages:

Speed: Pressure cooking can cut traditional cooking times by half or even more. Think pot roast in 60 minutes, unsoaked dried beans in 45 minutes, or a complete pasta dinner in 25 minutes.

Hands-off cooking: No more standing in front of the stove, adjusting the heat, and stirring constantly. With the Instant Pot, even a labor-intensive dish like risotto can cook almost entirely unattended.

Energy savings: With so many one-pot possibilities, you won't need multiple burners and the oven to get dinner on the table. This saves energy and helps keep your kitchen cool on the hottest summer days.

Healthier meal options: The speed and convenience of the Instant Pot means there's no need to order takeout or rely on prepackaged frozen dinners. You can cook healthier meals from scratch in about the same amount of time, all while controlling the ingredients you use.

Safety: The Instant Pot has multiple safety features. It automatically regulates the temperature and pressure with no oversight required. You can set it and walk away and know there's nothing to worry about.

Terms to Know

As you become familiar with your Instant Pot, there may be a few new terms.

Pressure release valve: The valve on the lid that controls the release of steam and pressure. In some models, it toggles between Sealing and Venting (in these recipes, it should always be set to Sealing). In the Ultra models, it's set to Sealing by default.

Sealing ring: The silicone ring that fits around the underside of the lid that seals the pot so pressure can build. It's crucial for this to be free of nicks or tears and placed correctly before the lid goes on.

Seal: When the pot comes to pressure, the lid will be sealed on the pot. Never try to remove a sealed lid.

Pot-in-pot cooking: The cooking method in which ingredients are placed in a bowl or other cooking dish, which is then placed on a trivet above water for steaming.

High pressure: The high-pressure setting is between 10.2 and 11.6 PSI (which produces cooking temperatures between 240°F and 245°F).

Low pressure: Available on all models except the Lux, low pressure is between 6 and 7 PSI (which produces a cooking temperature of 230°F).

Sauté: A setting to brown meats or vegetables or simmer sauces that can be set to low, medium, or high heat by pressing the Less or More buttons on the Duo model. Unless otherwise noted in the recipes, the Sauté setting is Normal by default.

Steam: The Steam setting heats faster and more constantly than the Pressure Cook or Manual settings, so the pot will come to pressure faster.

Pressure Cook/Manual: Depending on the model, there is either a Pressure Cook or Manual setting, used for customized cooking times.

Natural release: After cooking, this allows the pressure inside the pot to come down on its own, which can take 10 to 30 minutes depending on the contents.

Quick release: After cooking, the pressure can be released immediately by flipping the valve to Venting (or pressing the Quick Release button on the Ultra model).

Venting: The release valve setting that allows steam to escape. It's used to release pressure after cooking and in slow cooking and yogurt-making.

Keep warm: This default setting (which can be disabled) keeps food warm after cooking. In some models, the temperature is adjustable.

The Basic Steps of Instant Pot Cooking

Once you get the hang of using the Instant Pot, you'll be cooking like a pro in no time. Here's a rundown of some of the usual prep and cooking steps in the order in which you're likely to complete them.

1. **Precook ingredients.** With some recipes, you'll need to precook. What's wonderful is that you can do it all in the Instant Pot; there's no need for a skillet. First, you'll remove the lid and set it aside or conveniently hinge it on one of the side handles of the cooker base of the Instant Pot (yes, those handles can double as storage if you place the lid vertically into one of them). Then you'll brown meat or sauté vegetables using the Sauté function. If there are any bits of food stuck to the pot, you'll add a bit of liquid and scrape the pot to unstick them.

2. **Add liquid, the remaining ingredients, or both.** To pressure-steam foods like eggs, vegetables, or desserts, first you'll add water and the trivet or steaming basket. The food will go in a bowl or basket above the water. To pressure-cook foods directly, such as stews, pasta, and meat dishes, you'll put the ingredients right into the inner cooking pot, along with enough liquid to allow the pot to come to pressure.

3. **Lock the lid into place.** Once the lid is locked, you'll set the release valve to Sealing so that the pot can come to pressure.

4. **Select the cooking function, adjust the pressure, and input the cooking time.** Regardless of which cooking function you select, the pot will display a default time. You can adjust this using the [+] or [–] buttons to increase or decrease time. Depending on the model, you may or may not have to press a start button. The Ultra has one; other models do not. If there is no start button, a few seconds after you set the cooking time, the screen will display ON, which lets you know the pot is working to build pressure.

5. **Release pressure.** Once the cooking time finishes, you'll either let the pressure release naturally (meaning the pot cools down on its own), or you'll be instructed to do what is called a quick release by flipping the pressure release valve to Venting. In some instances, you'll let the pressure release naturally for a specified time and then flip the valve to Venting to quickly release the remaining steam.

6. **Finish the dish.** Some recipes will need finishing to bring the dish together. In this book, finishing instructions will have you thickening sauces, adding quick-cooking ingredients, or adjusting the seasoning.

ADJUSTING TO HIGH ALTITUDE

If you happen to live in an area of high altitude, you will need to adjust your cooking time to get the appropriate results, because water evaporates faster at higher altitudes. Most electric pressure cooker manufacturers recommend increasing the cooking time by 5 percent for every 1,000 feet over 2,000 feet of elevation. For example, if you live at 3,000 feet above sea level, multiply the cooking time by 1.05. If you live at 4,000 feet above sea level, you will need to multiply the cooking time by 1.10, and so on. There are two Instant Pot models, the Ultra and the Max, that will adjust the temperature for you—set the altitude, and the cooking time will be adjusted automatically.

Scaling Recipes Up and Down

Most of the recipes in this book yield 4 to 8 servings. But what if you want to double them for company or to have leftovers? What if you want to convert other recipes written for four or more servings down to two? When cooking under pressure, there are a few things to keep in mind.

Water: Regardless of scaling up or down, the one thing that will never change is the amount of water in the bottom of the pot when you're steaming food on the trivet or in a steamer basket. Whether you're steaming 3 ounces of green beans or 6 ounces, 4 eggs or 8 eggs, you'll use the same 1 cup of water.

Doubling: When you have a recipe that works, simply double everything. As long as the ingredients are cut the same, the cooking times generally won't change. The exception is when there's a very short cooking time. The extra ingredients may cause the pot to take longer to come to pressure, which can mean overcooking if the time is 5 minutes or less, such as the Garlicky Lemon Broccoli (page 41) or the Lemon-Ginger Asparagus (page 43). But mostly, it's easy to remember—double the ingredients, don't change the time. If you do find the dish is overcooked, subtract 1 minute from the pressure-cooking time, then test the ingredients to see if they are to your preference.

Scaling down: Scaling large recipes down is a bit trickier. In most cases, you can cut recipe ingredients in half to scale down, but there are a few things to look out for. One is liquid. With pressure cooking, you need liquid to boil to reach pressure. Depending on the other ingredients, you don't need much, but the total liquid should never be less than ¼ to ½ cup in order to avoid the Burn warning. Meats and vegetables release water as they cook, so you can easily get by with the smaller amount. Don't halve the oil or butter when it's used to sauté or brown ingredients. You'll need enough to cover the bottom of the pot, so you won't want to cut those ingredients past that point. As with doubling recipes, the cooking time will usually remain the same, but remember that with a smaller volume in the pot, it will take less time to come to pressure. You may occasionally need to increase the cooking time to account for that.

Supporting Equipment

Experienced Instant Pot users know that buying the pot is just the beginning. It's easy to go overboard buying accessories, but my list of essential equipment is short.

Baking dish: My go-to is a ceramic, straight-sided, 1-quart soufflé dish. Any metal, glass, or ceramic dish or bowl will work as long as it holds at least 3 cups. The diameter should be up to 7 inches for the 6-quart Instant Pot model and 6 inches or less for the 3-quart model.

Individual ramekins, custard cups, or small jars: Great for some breakfast and dessert recipes, they should hold 6 to 8 ounces with a diameter of about 4 inches for the 6-quart model or 3 inches for the 3-quart model. Silicone cups work as long as they are the right size and hold their shape. Larger ramekins (1½ cups) are also useful.

Springform pan: A 7-inch pan fits the 6-quart pot; for the 3-quart, it should be 6 inches or smaller. Alternatively, use a cake pan with a removable bottom. Mini springform pans (4 inches) can also be useful.

Steamer basket: I like the silicone models with locking handles. For these recipes, you don't need a big, deep basket; the shallow ones work fine.

Trivets: All Instant Pot models come with a trivet, but it might be worth buying one or two more. The trivets in the newer models have handles, but for older models, a trivet with handles is a good investment. There is even a silicone model. I also find it handy to have a tall trivet when cooking one food in a bowl over food in the bottom. It should be about 3 inches high.

Other useful tools include an immersion blender, food scale (for pasta and meat), sturdy tongs, fat separator, and silicone finger mitts for removing the inner pot or securing it while you stir ingredients.

Stocking Your Healthy Kitchen

We all know what it's like to look in your refrigerator or pantry only to find there is nothing to eat that is good for you. Having a kitchen well stocked with basic ingredients allows you to whip up a healthy meal at a moment's notice without having to make a separate trip to the grocery store.

Here are some of my favorite refrigerator and pantry staples, which I use repeatedly to create a variety of healthy, delicious dishes. Use this list as a starting place and then add or remove items based on your likes and dislikes.

REFRIGERATOR STAPLES

These common, store-bought fresh ingredients will serve as the backbone to many of the healthy recipes in this book.

Eggs: Eggs are essential in the kitchen for cooking or baking. They are a quick and easy way to get your daily protein and can be enjoyed at any time of the day.

Plain yogurt: Good for mixing into sauces and pureed soups for creaminess, plain yogurt can also be a healthier substitute for sour cream or mayonnaise.

Milk: Milk adds richness and depth to dishes and is often used in place of heavy cream to thicken sauces and soups. Unsweetened coconut and almond milk are good dairy-free milk substitutes.

Fresh fruits and vegetables: I always have a wide variety of fruits and vegetables on standby, including ones with long shelf lives, such as apples, sweet potatoes, and carrots, and ones that are best eaten fresh, like berries and leafy greens. Try to stick to seasonal fruits and vegetables since they generally taste better and are more affordable.

Fresh herbs: Cilantro, parsley, thyme, and rosemary are all-around amazing ingredients to add a pop of freshness to recipes. To keep the herbs fresh, wrap the bundle loosely in a damp paper towel, and store it in an airtight container or resealable bag in your crisper drawer.

Garlic: Fresh garlic is excellent to have around for flavoring savory dishes. Use fresh garlic cloves and peel them yourself, if possible, for the maximum flavor.

Cheese: Parmesan cheese adds a nutty flavor, and sharp Cheddar can be used in breakfast dishes and as a garnish for soup. Unless you're short on time or energy, opt to purchase them in block form instead of pre-grated or shredded for better taste.

PANTRY STAPLES

I always stock my pantry with staple ingredients I can use to create delicious and nutritious meals and snacks throughout the week.

Beans and lentils: Dried beans and lentils are inexpensive, extremely versatile, and have a long shelf life. Keep some canned beans on hand for when you're pressed for time.

Grains: Buy whole grains whenever you can. Oats, quinoa, and rice can be kept safely at room temperature for up to 6 months, if stored properly, or up to a year in the freezer, making them a smart choice to buy in bulk.

Cooking oils: Extra-virgin olive oil contains healthy fats and is rich in flavor. Pick a good-quality olive oil since the flavor will permeate everything you cook in it.

Dried herbs and spices: Cooking with aromatic ingredients such as chili powder, cinnamon, cumin, curry powder, and cayenne pepper elevates the flavor of dishes, and they can be used again and again.

Natural sweeteners: Honey and maple syrup add a touch of sweetness and flavor to both sweet and savory recipes.

Beef, chicken, and vegetable stock: Since the stock imparts flavors to recipes, be sure to choose one with a flavor base you like. Try to find ones that are low in sodium or, even better, sodium-free.

Healthy condiments: Condiments such as apple cider vinegar, Dijon mustard, reduced-sodium soy sauce, tahini, hot sauce, and salsa are flavor builders and can turn a dish from boring to exciting. These are used so often and in so many applications that they're always worth having.

HEALTHY SHOPPING ON A BUDGET

Shopping for healthy foods when you're on a budget doesn't have to be difficult. With some advance planning and strategy, you can eat balanced, wholesome meals without draining your wallet. Here are some easy and practical tips to help you shop wisely and save money.

Bulk bins are your friends: Most grocery stores have bulk bins where healthy grains, legumes, nuts, and baking ingredients are available at much lower prices than prepackaged. You can sometimes even find organic goods in bulk.

Choose in-season produce whenever possible: Fresh produce picked in season not only tastes better but also often promises the lowest prices, especially since stores always have sales on seasonal fruits and vegetables.

Buy quality frozen produce: When fruits and vegetables are out of season or too expensive to be purchased fresh, turn to the freezer aisle. Not only is frozen produce an excellent budget saver, but also it is convenient and ready to be used in recipes.

Shop with a list: Before grocery shopping for the week, plan your meals, take note of what you already have, and make a list for anything else. Shopping with a list helps you stick to buying what you need and prevents spontaneous purchases.

Stock up on staples: Pantry staples such as diced tomatoes, canned beans, and chicken stock have a long shelf life and are used in many recipes, so be sure to stock up whenever your grocery stores have these on sale.

Troubleshooting

I'm getting a "Burn" message. Why?

When a high temperature is detected at the bottom of the inner pot, its temperature sensor suspends heating. Early models show the message "ovHt" (overheat) and newer models show "burn." I think "overheat" is a more accurate warning, since it's not always, or even usually, burning food that causes the issue. The cause is likely a faulty seal or the sealing valve set to the Venting position rather than the Sealing position, either of which will keep the pot from coming to pressure and evaporate the liquid inside. Heating the pot empty before adding your ingredients can also cause the sensor to suspend heating, as can failing to scrape up any cooked bits of food from the sautéing process.

If you get the "burn" message, release any pressure, check the seal and valve, and check to see if there is food stuck to the bottom of the pot. Then—and this is important—let the pot cool off before starting again. The fastest way to do this is to take the inner pot out for a few minutes before resuming.

Why don't your recipes always include a cup of liquid?

There's virtually no loss of liquid in a pressure cooker, so it doesn't take much to create the steam necessary to keep the pot at pressure. Proteins and vegetables release liquid as they cook, so those recipes don't need a full cup to start. A pound of raw meat, for instance, will release more than ⅛ cup of liquid as it cooks—that's why pot roasts and pulled pork always have so much liquid at the end of the cooking process. Unless you are cooking foods that absorb water (grains, beans, or pasta), you don't need to start with the full cup needed when steaming foods. Too much liquid not only increases the time it takes for the pot to reach pressure, but also results in watery, under-seasoned food.

Why do you always use the Pressure Cook or Manual setting? Why not use the other cooking programs?

Although the preprogrammed settings can be handy, different models have different settings. The safest bet when I'm developing recipes is not to depend on a setting that's not universally available. I do occasionally use the Steam setting, since all models have that one. As you cook through the recipes, you should feel free to use the preprogrammed functions whenever appropriate.

Why does my pot take forever to come to pressure?

When you're waiting for that pin to come up and the countdown to start, it can seem like ages. The good news is you'll find that the time is not long when you're cooking small batches—smaller amounts take less time to heat up. When testing these recipes, the time to pressure was always less than 10 minutes—usually less than 8 minutes (a little longer for the Mini).

But all kinds of things can affect the process, like the temperature of your ingredients. If, with the recipes in this book, your pot hasn't started counting down within 12 minutes, something's probably wrong. Check the sealing ring and the valve.

Why do some of your recipes call for 0 minutes of pressure cooking? Is that a typo?

Remember that the pot begins heating immediately when it's turned on, so cooking begins well before the pot comes to pressure. And even with a quick release, you'll get an extra minute or so of cooking as the pressure releases. In some instances, that amount of cooking is all that's needed—as in the case of fast-cooking vegetables or shrimp—so 0 minutes is the right time to use.

The Recipes in This Book

The recipes in this book are all designed to be healthy and easy to prepare, even on a busy weeknight, using any size Instant Pot. They all include nutrition information, and most yield 4 to 8 servings. Entrées are 500 or fewer calories per serving; breakfasts are 300 or fewer calories per serving; snacks, sauces, and staples are fewer than 200 calories per serving; and sweet treats are fewer than 250 calories per serving. There will be no more guesswork about your calorie intake.

Although the recipes are designed to be healthy, I have also taken ingredient cost and availability into consideration. With that in mind, all the ingredients in this book are easily accessible at a reasonable price at any grocery store. To help with meal planning, many of these recipes include convenience labels indicating whether they are one-pot meals, can be made with 5 or fewer ingredients (excluding salt, pepper, water, and cooking oil or spray), are ready in less than 30 minutes, or are "worth the wait" if they take longer than 45 minutes to prepare from start to finish.

There are also a wide variety of recipes that cater to different types of dietary requirements. Look out for the following labels:

Gluten-free: These recipes do not have any grains that contain gluten, such as wheat, barley, or rye. That said, some ingredients, like canned vegetables, sauces, and seasonings, may contain trace amounts of gluten from processing, so if you have any doubts, be sure to check the ingredient label.

Dairy-free: These recipes do not contain any cow's milk products or ingredients, which makes them suitable for those who want to eliminate dairy products from their diet.

Vegetarian: These recipes do not contain meat, poultry, game, fish, shellfish, or by-products of animal slaughter. For this book, recipes labeled vegetarian may contain dairy products or eggs.

Vegan: These recipes do not contain animal products. The vegan label also encompasses dairy-free and vegetarian.

Whether you're at the beginning of your healthy eating journey or you're just looking for more inspiration, I hope you enjoy these recipes. I'm excited to share how easy it can be to make nourishing and satisfying dishes that the whole family will love. Let's get cooking!

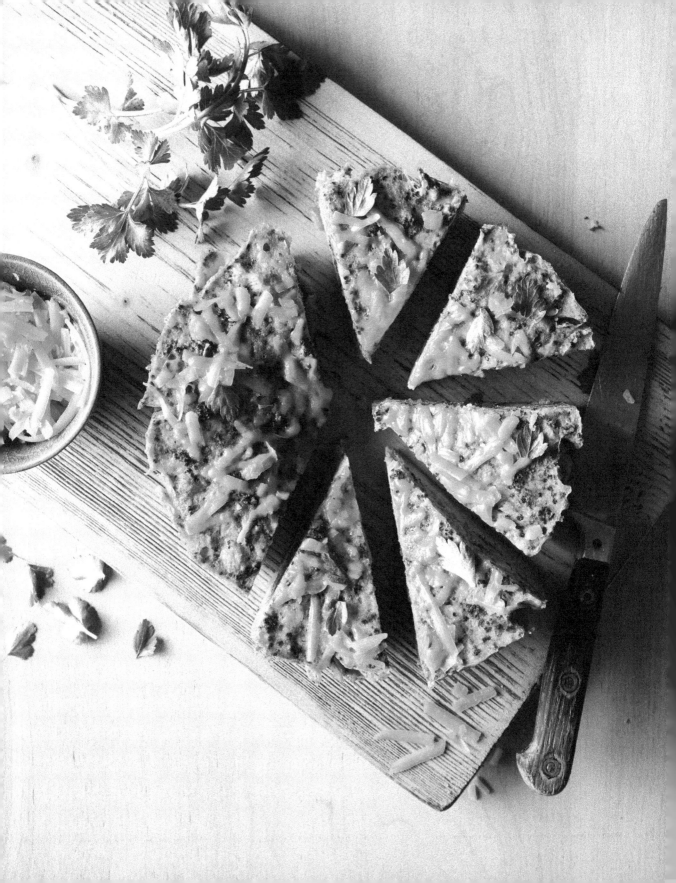

CHAPTER TWO

Breakfast and Brunch

BROCCOLI AND CHEDDAR CRUSTLESS QUICHE

Serves 6

Prep time: 10 minutes / **Pressure cook:** 30 minutes on High

Pressure release: Natural for 10 minutes, then Quick / **Total time:** 1 hour

 WORTH THE WAIT   5 OR FEWER INGREDIENTS

Making a quiche in the Instant Pot feels like a magic trick, especially when you don't want to use your oven. It's savory with just enough cheese to feel a bit decadent, so it's perfect for weekend brunch. The flour in the recipe isn't used to create a crust; rather, it gives the quiche some structure and makes it easy to slice.

Nonstick cooking spray, for coating the pan
1 cup water
8 large eggs
1 cup chopped broccoli florets
½ cup low-fat milk

½ cup whole-wheat flour
1½ cups shredded Cheddar cheese, divided
¼ teaspoon kosher salt
¼ teaspoon freshly ground black pepper
Fresh chopped parsley, for garnish (optional)

1. Grease a 6- to 7-inch soufflé or baking pan with cooking spray.

2. Place the trivet in the inner pot, then pour in the water.

3. If needed, make an aluminum foil sling (see page 29).

4. In a large bowl, whisk together the eggs, broccoli, milk, flour, 1 cup of cheese, the salt, and pepper.

5. Pour the mixture into the soufflé dish. Use the sling (if you made one) to lower the soufflé dish onto the trivet.

6. Lock the lid into place. Select Pressure Cook or Manual, and cook at High Pressure for 30 minutes.

7. After cooking, naturally release the pressure for 10 minutes, then quick release any remaining pressure.

8. Unlock and remove the lid. Use the sling to remove the soufflé dish.

9. Sprinkle the remaining ½ cup of cheese on top of the quiche.

10. Using a sharp knife, slice the quiche into 6 wedges.

11. Serve the quiche immediately, garnished with fresh parsley (if using), or place the quiche in an airtight container and refrigerate for up to 4 days.

Per Serving: Calories: 274; Fat: 19g; Protein: 17g; Carbohydrates: 10g; Fiber: 1.5g; Sugar: 1.5g; Sodium: 340mg

Soft-Boiled Eggs and Soldiers

Serves 4

Prep time: 5 minutes / **Pressure cook:** 6 minutes on Low

Pressure release: Quick / **Total time:** 15 minutes

 ONE-POT MEAL 5 OR FEWER INGREDIENTS QUICK

Kids and adults alike will love spending their morning dipping toast "soldiers" into runny egg yolks. The Instant Pot produces perfect soft-boiled eggs every time, and while they steam, you can toast and cut your bread. Breakfast is ready in 15 minutes flat.

---

1 cup water

4 large eggs

4 to 8 bread slices

1 to 2 tablespoons butter

1. Prepare the Instant Pot by pouring the water into the pot and placing the steam rack on top.

2. Place the eggs on the steam rack.

3. Lock the lid into place. Select Pressure Cook or Manual, and cook at Low Pressure for 6 minutes.

4. While the eggs cook, toast and butter the bread. Cut into 1-inch strips.

5. After cooking, quick release the pressure. Carefully remove the eggs, and place in egg cups.

6. Using a spoon, tap around the top of each egg in a circle. Remove the top circle of shell and the section of egg along with it, exposing the runny yolk.

7. Serve the eggs with the toast for dunking.

❖ **Flavor Boost:** Eggs and soldiers is a popular British breakfast, and the toast is often spread with Marmite, or in Australia, Vegemite.

Per Serving (1 egg + 2 slices bread): Calories: 252; Fat: 13g; Protein: 10g; Carbohydrates: 20g; Fiber: 1g; Sugar: 3g; Sodium: 302mg

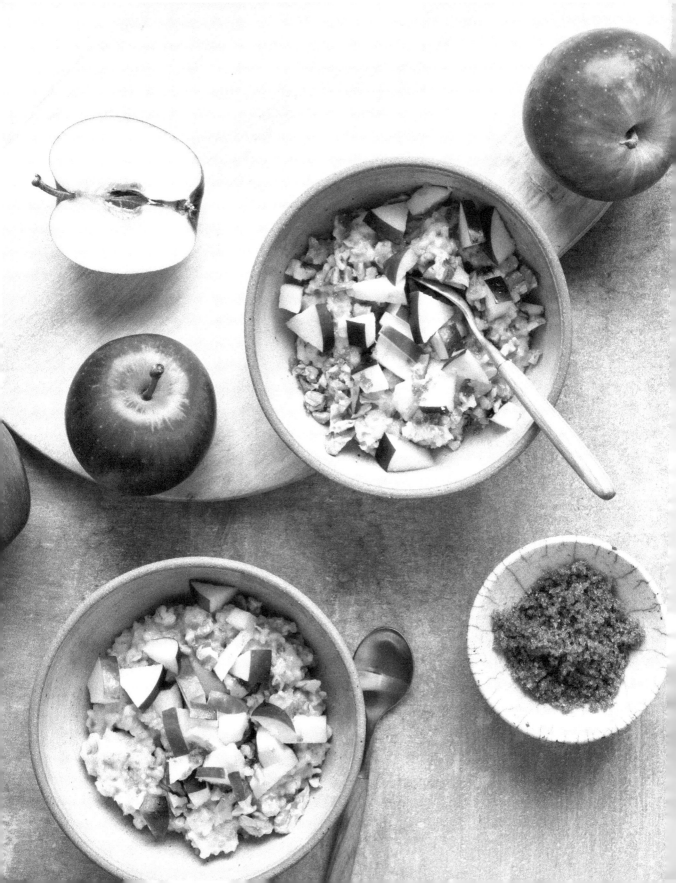

Apple-Cinnamon Oatmeal

Serves 4

Prep time: 5 minutes / **Pressure cook:** 7 minutes on High

Pressure release: Natural for 10 minutes, then Quick / **Total time:** 30 minutes

 ONE-POT MEAL   5 OR FEWER INGREDIENTS   QUICK

Heart-healthy steel-cut oatmeal cooks perfectly in no time in the pressure cooker, and cinnamon and apple make this an autumn morning must. If you've never tried steel-cut oats, they're the chewier, healthier cousin of instant oats. If you're gluten intolerant, be sure to buy oats that are labeled as gluten-free. Top with chopped walnuts or pecans for a bit of protein and crunch.

3 tablespoons unsalted butter

1 cup steel-cut oats

2½ cups water

1 large apple, cored, peeled, and chopped, plus more for garnish

1 tablespoon brown sugar, plus more (optional) for serving

1 teaspoon ground cinnamon

¼ teaspoon kosher salt

1. Preheat the Instant Pot by selecting Sauté. Once hot, toss in the butter, and melt.

2. Add the oats, and stir. Cook for 2 minutes.

3. Add the water, apple, sugar, cinnamon, and salt. Stir.

4. Lock the lid into place. Select Pressure Cook or Manual, and cook at High Pressure for 7 minutes.

5. After cooking, naturally release the pressure for 10 minutes, then quick release any remaining pressure.

6. Unlock and remove the lid. The oatmeal will continue to thicken as it cools.

7. Serve the oatmeal topped with chopped apple. If desired, sprinkle with more brown sugar.

✿ **Variation Tip:** For stronger apple flavor, replace up to 1 cup of the water with apple cider, and omit the brown sugar.

Per Serving: Calories: 188; Fat: 9.5g; Protein: 9g; Carbohydrates: 17g; Fiber: 3.5g; Sugar: 4g; Sodium: 218mg

POBLANO-SWEET POTATO HASH

Serves 4 to 6

Prep time: 2 hours / **Pressure cook:** 2 minutes on High; 13 minutes on Sauté Low
Pressure release: Quick / **Total time:** 2 hours 20 minutes

  WORTH THE WAIT

This hash is worth the extra step of preparing the tofu separately; when you combine it with the sweet potatoes and peppers, you end up with multiple delicious textures and a more complex flavor. It's also important to let the liquid press out of the tofu to ensure it can get nice and crispy.

---

2 medium sweet potatoes, peeled and cut into large dice
1 cup water
2 tablespoons extra-virgin olive oil, divided
1 (14-ounce) package extra-firm tofu, pressed for at least 2 hours, then crumbled in a food processor
1 teaspoon ground turmeric

½ teaspoon smoked paprika
½ teaspoon kosher salt
1 small yellow onion, diced
1 bell pepper, any color, cored and diced
2 poblano peppers, roasted, cored, and diced
2 garlic cloves, minced
1½ teaspoons Montreal chicken seasoning

1. In the inner pot, combine the sweet potatoes and water.

2. Lock the lid into place. Select Pressure Cook or Manual, and cook at High Pressure for 2 minutes.

3. After cooking, quick release the pressure.

4. Unlock and remove the lid. Pour the contents of the inner pot into a colander or steamer basket to drain. Return the inner pot to the Instant Pot, and set the sweet potatoes aside.

5. Select Sauté, and add 1 tablespoon of oil to the inner pot.

6. Once the oil is hot, add the tofu, turmeric, paprika, and salt. Cook, stirring often, for 4 to 5 minutes, or until the tofu gets a little crispy. Remove from the pot and set aside.

7. To the inner pot, add the remaining 1 tablespoon of oil, the onion, and bell pepper. Cook for 2 to 3 minutes.

8. Add the poblano peppers, garlic, and Montreal chicken seasoning. Cook for 1 minute.

9. Add the sweet potatoes back to the pot. Cook, stirring frequently, for 2 to 3 minutes.

10. Press Cancel, and stir in the tofu. Mix well to combine, and serve warm.

♻ **Ingredient Tip:** Try roasting your own poblano peppers! Rub them with oil, and put them on a baking sheet. Roast in a 425°F oven, turning occasionally, for 30 to 45 minutes, or until the skin is charred on all sides. Remove from the oven. Using tongs, put the peppers in a bowl, and cover with plastic wrap. Let sit for 15 minutes. Run the peppers under cold water, and rub off the skins.

Per Serving: Calories: 188; Fat: 9.5g; Protein: 9g; Carbohydrates: 17g; Fiber: 3.5g; Sugar: 4g; Sodium: 218mg

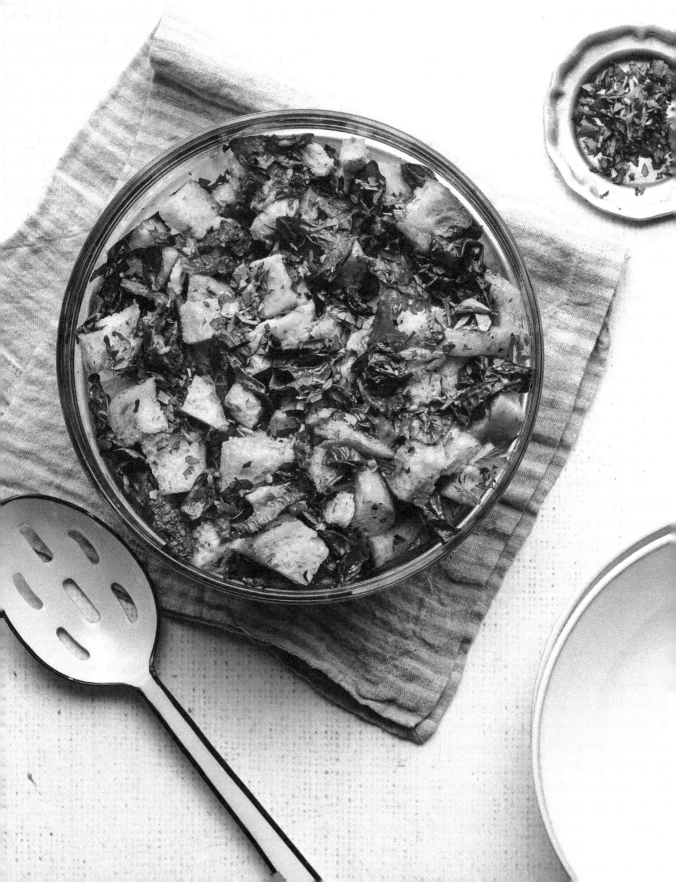

SAVORY STRATA

Serves 6

Prep time: 15 minutes, plus 2 hours to chill / **Pressure cook:** 25 minutes on High

Pressure release: Natural for 10 minutes, then Quick / **Total time:** 1 hour, plus 2 hours to chill

 WORTH THE WAIT

Throw this strata together before bed and put it in the electric pressure cooker the next day, and you've got a delicious one-pot dish that's perfect for guests or weekend brunch. It's also a great way to use up some vegetables, cheese, or bread.

1 cup low-sodium vegetable stock	1 bunch Swiss chard, stemmed and chopped
4 large eggs	1/3 cup oil-packed sun-dried tomatoes, chopped
1½ teaspoons Italian seasoning	1/3 cup grated parmesan cheese
½ teaspoon kosher salt	Nonstick cooking spray, for coating
¼ teaspoon freshly ground black pepper	¼ cup water
¼ teaspoon red pepper flakes	1/3 cup chopped fresh parsley (optional)
4 cups cubed sourdough bread	

1. In a large bowl, beat together the stock, eggs, Italian seasoning, salt, pepper, and red pepper flakes.

2. Mix in the bread, chard, tomatoes, and cheese. Cover, and refrigerate for 2 hours or up to overnight.

3. Grease a 2-quart soufflé dish or 7-cup round glass container with cooking spray.

4. Transfer the egg mixture to the dish. Cover tightly with aluminum foil, and place on a steam rack.

5. Pour the water into the inner pot, then carefully place the steam rack and dish in the pot.

6. Lock the lid into place. Select Pressure Cook or Manual, and cook at High Pressure for 25 minutes.

7. After cooking, naturally release the pressure for 10 minutes, then quick release any remaining pressure.

8. Unlock and remove the lid. Carefully remove the steam rack and dish.

9. Garnish with the parsley (if using), and serve.

❖ **Variation Tip:** Swap out the Swiss chard and parmesan for whatever you like! Spinach or kale would work beautifully and pairs nicely with feta, goat cheese, Cheddar, or Manchego.

Per Serving: Calories: 270; Carbohydrates: 40g; Fat: 6g; Fiber: 2g; Protein: 14g; Sugar: 2g; Sodium: 700mg

Banana Bread

Serves 8

Prep time: 10 minutes / **Pressure cook:** 55 minutes on High

Pressure release: Natural for 10 minutes, then Quick / **Total time:** 1 hour 25 minutes

 WORTH THE WAIT

If bananas I have get too ripe, I let them get even more brown and use them to make banana bread. In fact, the darker the banana is, the sweeter and more flavorful it gets. Baking in the Instant Pot produces incredibly moist and delicious banana bread.

1½ cups water

¾ cup packed brown sugar

4 tablespoons (½ stick) unsalted butter, at room temperature

¼ cup unsweetened applesauce

3 medium ripe bananas, mashed

2 large eggs, beaten

1 teaspoon vanilla extract

2 cups whole-wheat flour

1 teaspoon baking soda

1 teaspoon ground cinnamon

½ teaspoon kosher salt

Nonstick cooking spray, for coating the pan

1. Prepare the Instant Pot by pouring the water into the pot and placing the steam rack on top.

2. In a large bowl, mix together the sugar, butter, and applesauce.

3. Add the bananas, eggs, and vanilla. Stir until well blended.

4. In a medium bowl, combine the flour, baking soda, cinnamon, and salt.

5. Add the dry ingredients to the wet ingredients, and mix until just combined.

6. Grease a 7-inch cake pan with cooking spray.

7. Pour the batter into the prepared pan. Cover tightly with aluminum foil, leaving room for expansion.

8. Place the cake pan on the steam rack.

9. Lock the lid into place. Select Pressure Cook or Manual, and cook at High Pressure for 55 minutes.

10. After cooking, naturally release the pressure for 10 minutes, then quick release any remaining pressure.

11. Unlock the lid, and carefully remove the cake pan using the handles. Remove the foil, and allow the bread to cool in the pan for 10 minutes before serving.

Per Serving: Calories: 216; Carbohydrates: 35g; Fat: 8g; Fiber: 3g; Protein: 4g; Sugar: 20g; Sodium: 370mg

Cinnamon-Raisin French Toast Bake

Serves 6

Prep time: 10 minutes / **Pressure cook:** 15 minutes on High

Pressure release: Quick / **Total time:** 35 minutes

This breakfast casserole is a handy way to use up old bread and has all the flavor and texture of French toast plus a little cinnamon spice. For a crisp top, sprinkle with sugar and slide under the broiler for a few minutes at the end.

1½ cups water

1 teaspoon butter

3 large eggs

1 cup whole or low-fat milk

2 tablespoons maple syrup, plus more
    for serving

1 teaspoon vanilla extract

3 cups cubed (¾-inch) stale or lightly toasted
    cinnamon-raisin bread

1 teaspoon sugar (optional)

1. Prepare the Instant Pot by pouring the water into the pot and placing the steam rack on top.

2. Butter a 6- to 7-inch soufflé or baking pan. (If your pan doesn't have handles, make a sling for it before putting it into the pot. See the Cooking Tip for instructions.)

3. In a large bowl, whisk together the eggs, milk, maple syrup, and vanilla.

4. Add the bread, and let sit, stirring once or twice, for 5 minutes.

5. Pour the mixture into the pan, and push down to submerge the bread if needed.

6. Place the pan on the steam rack.

7. Lock the lid into place. Select Pressure Cook or Manual, and cook at High Pressure for 15 minutes.

8. After cooking, quick release the pressure. Be sure to remove the lid carefully and quickly so that condensation doesn't drip onto the French toast.

9. Carefully remove the pan using a sling or handles. If a crispy top is desired, sprinkle with the sugar, and broil for 3 to 5 minutes.

❖ **Cooking Tip:** If your dish or steam rack doesn't have handles, create a sling with a piece of aluminum foil, folded in half twice, that's long enough to go under the dish and stick up 6 inches on each side, creating "handles."

Per Serving: Calories: 210; Fat: 5.5g; Protein: 7g; Carbohydrates: 34g; Fiber: 1g; Sugar: 19g; Sodium: 176mg

POACHED EGGS

Serves 4

Prep time: 10 minutes / **Pressure cook:** 4 minutes on Sauté High

Pressure release: None / **Total time:** 15 minutes

 5 OR FEWER INGREDIENTS   QUICK

Cracking an egg into a cup and steaming it is a great way to cook eggs, but it's not poaching. But you *can* use your Instant Pot to poach eggs. Use the Sauté function to heat the poaching liquid, and with a few tips, a couple of pieces of equipment, and a little practice, you'll be able to produce gorgeous, perfectly cooked poached eggs.

8 cups water

2 tablespoons kosher salt

1 tablespoon distilled white vinegar

4 large eggs

Buttered toast or English muffins, for serving (optional)

1. Pour the water into the inner pot, and add the salt and vinegar. (The combination of acid and salt acts on the alkaline whites and brings the eggs to the surface of the water as they cook so they cook evenly.) Line a plate with paper towels.

2. Select Sauté, and adjust to More for high heat. As the water heats, stir to dissolve the salt. Heat the water to just below the boiling point—between 200°F and 205°F.

3. Place a small strainer over a custard cup or ramekin. Crack an egg into the strainer, and let sit for a couple of minutes to drain off the thin egg whites. (This makes a neater-looking poached egg, since it's the thin whites that fly around in the water.) Gently tip the egg in the strainer into a new custard cup. Repeat with the remaining eggs, placing each egg in a separate cup.

4. When the water has heated, tip the eggs one at a time from the cup into the water, spacing the eggs evenly and keeping track of the order you put them in the water. Cook each egg for 3 to 4 minutes. Press Cancel to stop cooking.

5. Using a large, slotted spoon, remove the eggs to the prepared plate. Drain briefly.

6. To serve, place the eggs in cups or on buttered toast (if using).

❖ **Ingredient Tip:** If you make your toast while the water is heating and the eggs are draining, you can keep it on a rack in a low oven or warming drawer while you cook the eggs. That way, you'll have warm toast and hot eggs at the same time.

Per Serving: Calories: 71; Fat: 4.5g; Protein: 6g; Carbohydrates: 0g; Fiber: 0g; Sugar: 0g; Sodium: 239mg

QUINOA BREAKFAST PORRIDGE

Serves 4

Prep time: 5 minutes / **Pressure cook:** 2 minutes on High

Pressure release: Natural for 10 minutes, then Quick / **Total time:** 30 minutes

 ONE-POT MEAL   5 OR FEWER INGREDIENTS   QUICK

If you've only used quinoa in savory recipes, try this new way to enjoy it for breakfast! Cooking quinoa in the Instant Pot is quick and easy and results in a creamy consistency every time. Not only is this warm quinoa porridge a delicious and comforting way to start the day, but also it gives you the added boost of protein to get you through your morning.

---

1 cup quinoa, rinsed and drained

3 cups unsweetened vanilla almond milk, divided

¼ teaspoon kosher salt

1 cup raspberries

¼ cup sliced almonds

¼ cup maple syrup

1. In the inner pot, combine the quinoa, 2 cups of almond milk, and the salt.

2. Lock the lid into place. Select Pressure Cook or Manual, and cook at High Pressure for 2 minutes.

3. After cooking, naturally release the pressure for 10 minutes, then quick release any remaining pressure.

4. Fluff the quinoa with a fork. Stir in the remaining 1 cup of almond milk.

5. Serve the quinoa porridge topped with the raspberries, almonds, and maple syrup.

♻ **Ingredient Tip:** This dish is perfect for meal prepping. Make a big batch, refrigerate in an airtight container, and reheat individual portions throughout the week. Since quinoa thickens slightly as it cools, add a splash of water or milk before reheating for a thinner consistency.

Per Serving: Calories: 288; Carbohydrates: 47g; Fat: 8g; Fiber: 7g; Protein: 8g; Sugar: 13g; Sodium: 287mg

FLORENTINE EGG BITES

Serves 7

Prep time: 5 minutes / **Pressure cook:** 10 minutes on High
Pressure release: Quick / **Total time:** 25 minutes

 5 OR FEWER INGREDIENTS   QUICK

For a nutritious bite in the morning, look no further. These egg bites have everything you need to fuel your day. They're light and fluffy, perfectly flavorful, and make for a great grab-and-go breakfast. This recipe is very versatile, so feel free to experiment with your favorite add-ins to create your own tasty egg bites.

1½ cups water
4 large eggs
⅓ cup cottage cheese
¼ cup grated parmesan cheese
¼ teaspoon kosher salt

¼ teaspoon freshly ground black pepper
Nonstick cooking spray, for coating the
    egg mold
½ roasted red pepper, chopped
½ cup fresh baby spinach, chopped

1. Prepare the Instant Pot by pouring the water into the pot and placing the steam rack on top.

2. Put the eggs, cottage cheese, parmesan cheese, salt, and pepper in a blender. Process for about 30 seconds, or until smooth.

3. Grease a silicone egg mold with cooking spray.

4. Divide the red pepper and baby spinach evenly between the compartments of the silicone mold, pour in the egg mixture, and tightly cover with aluminum foil.

5. Place the egg mold on the steam rack.

6. Lock the lid into place. Select Pressure Cook or Manual, and cook at High Pressure for 10 minutes.

7. After cooking, quick release the pressure. Remove the lid, and carefully remove the mold using the handles.

8. Let the egg bites cool for 2 minutes before releasing them one by one from the mold. Serve warm.

❧ **Substitution Tip:** To lower the cholesterol and calories in these egg bites, replace the 4 whole eggs with 8 egg whites or 1 cup egg substitute.

Per Serving: Calories: 74; Fat: 5g; Protein: 6g; Carbohydrates: 1g; Fiber: 0.5g; Sugar: 0.5g; Sodium: 196mg

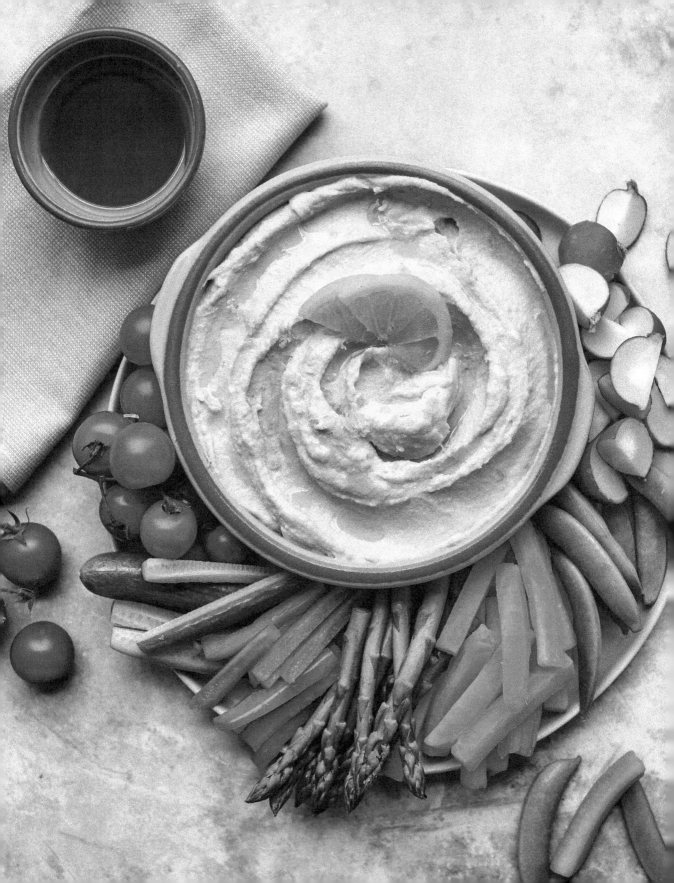

CHAPTER THREE

Snacks and Sides

HUMMUS

Makes 1½ cups

Prep time: 5 minutes, plus 8 hours to soak / **Pressure cook:** 3 minutes on High

Pressure release: Natural / **Total time:** 8 hours 15 minutes

 5 OR FEWER INGREDIENTS

2 tablespoons plus ¼ teaspoon kosher
  salt, divided
2 quarts water, divided
4 ounces dried chickpeas
1 teaspoon plus 2 tablespoons extra-virgin olive
  oil, divided
1 tablespoon freshly squeezed lemon juice, plus
  more as needed

1 tablespoon tahini (optional)
¼ teaspoon ground cumin, plus more as needed
1 garlic clove, minced
2 or 3 tablespoons ice water

1. In a large bowl, dissolve 1 tablespoon of salt in 1 quart of water.

2. Add the chickpeas, and soak at room temperature for 8 to 24 hours.
    Drain and rinse.

3. Put the chickpeas and 1 teaspoon of olive oil in the inner pot. Stir to coat.

4. Add the remaining 1 quart of water and 1 tablespoon of salt.

5. Lock the lid into place. Select Pressure Cook or Manual, and cook at High
    Pressure for 3 minutes.

6. After cooking, naturally release the pressure.

7. Unlock and remove the lid. Drain the chickpeas, then transfer to a food processor.

8. Add the remaining 2 tablespoons of olive oil, remaining ¼ teaspoon of salt, the
    lemon juice, tahini (if using), cumin, and garlic. Process until a coarse paste
    forms. Stop the machine several times to scrape down the sides; don't worry if
    the mixture contains a few chunks, but it should be mostly smooth.

9. Remove the cover from the feed tube, and with the motor running, pour in
    2 tablespoons of ice water. Process until the puree is smooth, adding another
    tablespoon of water if necessary.

10. Cover the hummus with plastic wrap so it doesn't dry out. Store in the refrigera-
    tor for up to 1 week.

Per Serving (¼ cup): Calories: 116; Fat: 6.5g; Protein: 4g; Carbohydrates: 12g; Fiber: 3.5g; Sugar: 3g;
Sodium: 163mg

Spinach-Artichoke Dip

Serves 8

Prep time: 20 minutes / **Pressure cook:** 5 minutes on Sauté; 7 minutes on High
Pressure release: Quick / **Total time:** 40 minutes

This creamy dip is perfect for parties and get-togethers. If by chance some leftover dip remains after a gathering, it can also be used as a sauce for pastas or a spread for sandwiches. This dip is also perfect for making in bulk because it stores well in the refrigerator and freezer.

---

2 teaspoons extra-virgin olive oil
1 small yellow onion, diced
2 garlic cloves, minced
8 ounces fresh spinach, coarsely chopped
   (about 1 bunch)
½ teaspoon kosher salt
1 teaspoon freshly ground black pepper

5 ounces cream cheese
1 (8½-ounce) can water-packed artichoke
   hearts, drained and quartered
⅓ cup heavy cream
⅓ cup water
Chips or sliced vegetables, for serving

1. Select Sauté, and pour the oil into the inner pot.

2. Once the oil is hot, add the onion and garlic. Sauté for 1 minute.

3. Add the spinach, salt, and pepper. Sauté for 2 to 3 minutes, or until the spinach has wilted.

4. Add the cream cheese, artichokes, cream, and water. Mix thoroughly.

5. Lock the lid into place. Select Pressure Cook or Manual, and cook at High Pressure for 7 minutes.

6. After cooking, quick release the pressure.

7. Unlock and remove the lid. Stir the dip, then leave to cool in the Instant Pot with the lid off. Transfer to a serving bowl.

8. Serve the dip with chips or sliced vegetables.

❖ **Ingredient Tip:** Instead of fresh spinach, you can use about 5 ounces (⅔ cup) frozen spinach, which is less expensive. Be sure to thaw it to room temperature before using. Cook time and pressure remain the same when thawed.

Per Serving (without dippers): Calories: 129; Fat: 11g; Protein: 3g; Carbohydrates: 6g; Fiber: 1g; Sugar: 1.5g; Sodium: 280mg

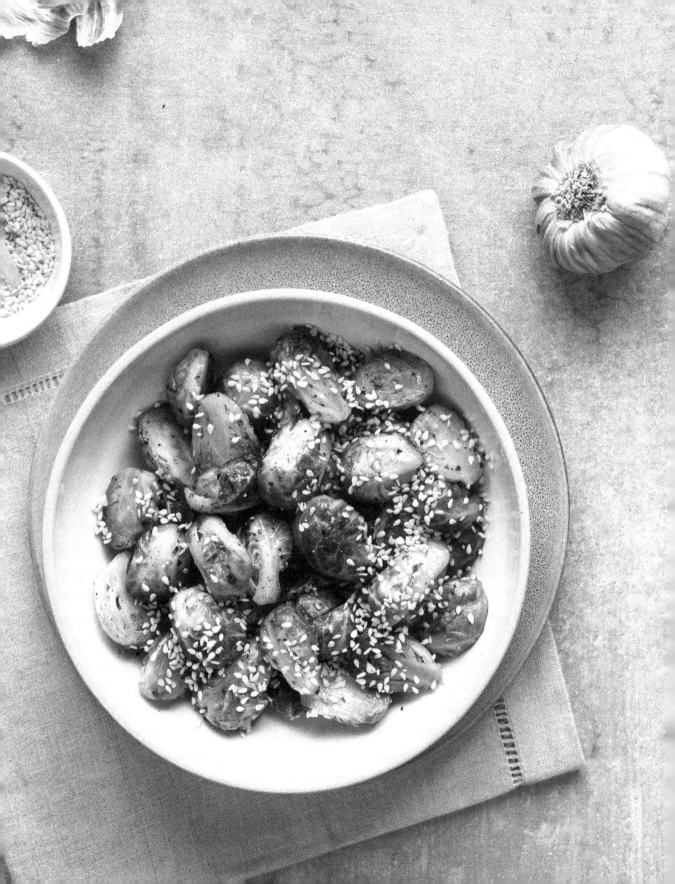

BALSAMIC BRUSSELS SPROUTS

Serves 4

Prep time: 15 minutes / **Steam:** 1 minute / **Pressure cook:** 3 minutes on Sauté

Pressure release: Quick / **Total time:** 30 minutes

 5 OR FEWER INGREDIENTS   QUICK

Get your daily dose of valuable nutrients with these delicious Brussels sprouts. The balsamic vinegar and sesame seeds add balance and texture—a hint of sweet and tangy flavor, plus that extra crunch. It's a perfect side dish for any meal.

---

1 pound Brussels sprouts, trimmed and halved lengthwise

1 cup water

1 tablespoon extra-virgin olive oil

2 garlic cloves, minced

1 tablespoon balsamic vinegar

1 teaspoon kosher salt

½ teaspoon freshly ground black pepper

1 tablespoon toasted sesame seeds

1. Put the Brussels sprouts in a steamer basket.

2. Pour the water into the inner pot, and place the trivet inside. Place the basket on the trivet.

3. Lock the lid into place. Select Steam, and set the time to 1 minute.

4. After cooking, quick release the pressure.

5. Unlock and remove the lid. Using tongs, carefully transfer the Brussels sprouts to a serving plate. Discard the water, and wipe the inner pot dry.

6. Select Sauté, and pour the oil into the inner pot.

7. Once the oil is hot, add the garlic, and sauté for 1 minute.

8. Add the Brussels sprouts, vinegar, salt, and pepper. Sauté for 2 minutes. Press Cancel to stop cooking.

9. Sprinkle with the sesame seeds, and serve hot.

♻ **Variation Tip:** Instead of Brussels sprouts, use asparagus, broccoli, or green beans, or to save time, just leave the Brussels sprouts whole and add an extra minute to the pressure-cooking time.

Per Serving: Calories: 97; Fat: 4.5g; Protein: 4g; Carbohydrates: 12g; Fiber: 4.5g; Sugar: 3g; Sodium: 314mg

POTATOES WITH GREENS

Serves 4

Prep time: 15 minutes / **Pressure cook:** 7 minutes on High

Pressure release: Quick / **Total time:** 35 minutes

 ONE-POT MEAL 5 OR FEWER INGREDIENTS

There are many different varieties of potatoes, but I find that small, waxy types work best in this dish. This is because they are less starchy and retain their shape and structure better in the Instant Pot. Look for mini or small potatoes that are one bite when cut in half. Waxy potato varieties include new potatoes, red bliss, fingerlings, and blue or red potatoes, to name a few. Other hearty greens, such as collard greens or mustard greens, can be used in place of the kale if preferred.

---

1 teaspoon extra-virgin olive oil

5 garlic cloves, sliced

2 bunches kale, stemmed and chopped

1½ pounds small new potatoes, skin-on and halved

1 cup water or low-sodium vegetable stock

2 tablespoons freshly squeezed lemon juice

1 teaspoon kosher salt

¼ teaspoon freshly ground black pepper

1. Select Sauté, and pour the oil into the inner pot.

2. Once the oil is hot, add the garlic, and sauté for about 30 seconds, or until fragrant.

3. Add the kale, potatoes, water, lemon juice, salt, and pepper. Mix well.

4. Lock the lid into place. Select Pressure Cook or Manual, and cook at High Pressure for 7 minutes.

5. After cooking, quick release the pressure.

6. Unlock and remove the lid. Serve warm.

❖ **Ingredient Tip:** Pre-chopped kale can be used to cut down on prep time.

Per Serving: Calories: 180; Fat: 2g; Protein: 9g; Carbohydrates: 39g; Fiber: 7g; Sugar: 6g; Sodium: 320mg

GARLICKY LEMON BROCCOLI

Serves 2 to 4

Prep time: 5 minutes / **Pressure cook:** 0 minutes on High

Pressure release: Quick / **Total time:** 10 minutes

 5 OR FEWER INGREDIENTS QUICK

This is a healthy side dish with a mild flavor that lets your main dish shine. Sometimes simple is best! And broccoli is always a winner in my book. Did you know broccoli was first cultivated in Italy during ancient Roman times, becoming common in England and America in the 1700s? I can imagine the pilgrims eating broccoli, but I'm sure theirs wasn't prepared with lemon or garlic! Those poor pilgrims never knew what they were missing.

1 cup water

4 garlic cloves, coarsely chopped

6 cups chopped broccoli

Grated zest and juice of 1 lemon, divided

½ teaspoon kosher salt

1. In the inner pot, combine the water and garlic.

2. Put the broccoli in a steamer basket, and put the basket into the inner pot.

3. Pour the lemon juice over the broccoli so it runs down into the water.

4. Lock the lid into place. Select Pressure Cook or Manual, and cook at High Pressure for 0 minutes.

5. After cooking, quick release the pressure.

6. Unlock and remove the lid. Remove the broccoli.

7. Sprinkle the salt and lemon zest over the broccoli. Stir well.

Per Serving: Calories: 70; Fat: 0.5g; Protein: 5g; Carbohydrates: 14g; Fiber: 5g; Sugar: 3.5g; Sodium: 246mg

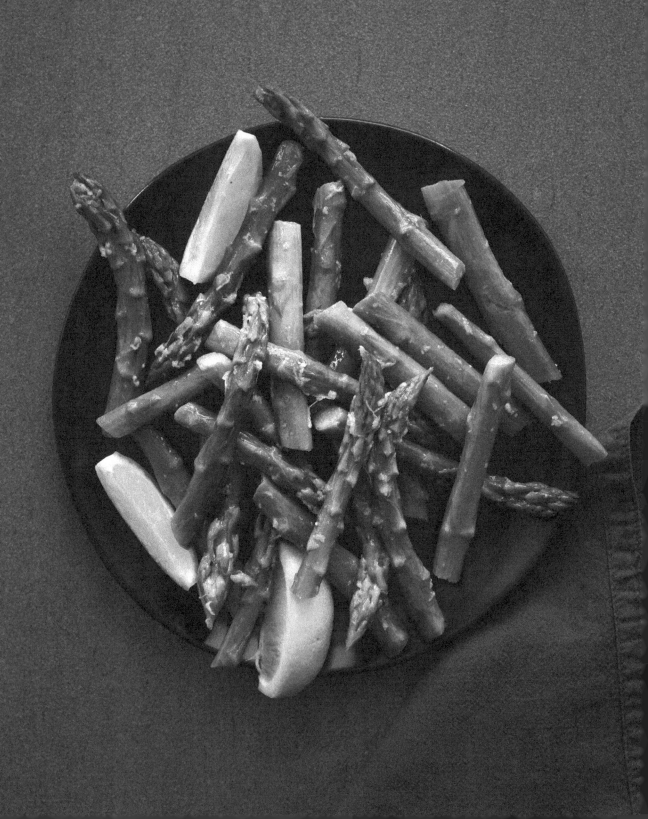

Lemon-Ginger Asparagus

Serves 4 to 6

Prep time: 5 minutes / **Pressure cook:** 0 minutes on Low

Pressure release: Quick / **Total time:** 10 minutes

 5 OR FEWER INGREDIENTS **QUICK**

This dish just screams springtime to me—the light, bright flavors create a delicious side dish. You'll notice I've listed a range of measurements for the seasonings. That's because ginger and lemon can quickly overwhelm the asparagus if you're not careful. I recommend starting with ½ teaspoon of each and tasting after adding the asparagus. It's easy to add more, but there's no turning back if you add too much.

1 bunch asparagus, tough ends removed, halved if remaining pieces are longer than 4 inches

1 cup water

2 tablespoons extra-virgin olive oil

1½ teaspoons to 1 tablespoon freshly squeezed lemon juice

½ to 1 teaspoon kosher salt

½ to ¾ teaspoon peeled and grated fresh ginger

1. Put the asparagus in a steamer basket, and put the basket into the Instant Pot.

2. Add the water.

3. Lock the lid into place. Select Pressure Cook or Manual, and cook at Low Pressure for 0 minutes.

4. In a medium serving bowl, stir together the oil, lemon juice, ½ teaspoon of salt, and ½ teaspoon of ginger.

5. After cooking, quick release the pressure.

6. Unlock and remove the lid. Add the asparagus to the bowl. Toss to combine. Taste, and add the remaining lemon juice, ginger, or both as needed.

Per Serving: Calories: 67; Fat: 5.5g; Protein: 2g; Carbohydrates: 4g; Fiber: 1g; Sugar: 1.5g; Sodium: 170mg

Cilantro-Lime Rice

Serves 4

Prep time: 5 minutes / **Pressure cook:** 3 minutes on High

Pressure release: Natural for 10 minutes, then Quick / **Total time:** 25 minutes

  5 OR FEWER INGREDIENTS   QUICK

Sometimes you just need an easy side dish to complete your meal, and thankfully, making rice in the Instant Pot couldn't be simpler. This cilantro-lime rice has bright, fresh flavor and pairs well with Mexican-inspired dishes like tacos, fajitas, or enchiladas. To make a big batch for meal prep, double the recipe, and keep the cook time the same.

---

1 cup long-grain white rice, rinsed well and drained

1¼ cups water

1 teaspoon extra-virgin olive oil

1 teaspoon kosher salt

½ cup chopped fresh cilantro

1 tablespoon freshly squeezed lime juice

1 teaspoon grated lime zest

1. In the inner pot, combine the rice, water, oil, and salt.

2. Lock the lid into place. Select Pressure Cook or Manual, and cook at High Pressure for 3 minutes.

3. After cooking, naturally release the pressure for 10 minutes, then quick release any remaining pressure.

4. Unlock and remove the lid. Fluff the rice with a fork.

5. Add the cilantro, lime juice, and lime zest. Toss until well mixed. Serve warm, refrigerate in a sealed container for up to 4 days, or freeze for up to 3 months.

❖ **Variation Tip:** You can substitute brown rice for white rice; just increase the cooking time to 22 minutes.

Per Serving: Calories: 180; Fat: 1.5g; Protein: 3g; Carbohydrates: 37g; Fiber: 0.5g; Sugar: 0g; Sodium: 283mg

Deviled Eggs

Serves 6

Prep time: 5 minutes / **Pressure cook:** 8 minutes on High
Pressure release: Natural for 5 minutes, then Quick / **Total time:** 25 minutes

 5 OR FEWER INGREDIENTS   QUICK

Here's a lightened-up version of the classic favorite. Typically, deviled eggs are made with mayonnaise, but I replaced part of the mayonnaise with tangy and thick Greek yogurt, which is higher in protein and has fewer calories. They taste creamy and decadent with less than 90 calories per serving, so there is no need to feel guilty about this delicious snack.

---

1 cup water
6 large eggs
2 tablespoons 2 percent plain Greek yogurt
1 tablespoon light mayonnaise
1 teaspoon Dijon mustard

¼ teaspoon Hot Sauce (page 131) or your
   favorite hot sauce brand
Kosher salt
Freshly ground black pepper
Smoked paprika, for garnish (optional)

1. Prepare the Instant Pot by pouring the water into the pot and placing the steam rack on top.

2. Arrange the eggs on top of the rack.

3. Lock the lid into place. Select Pressure Cook or Manual, and cook at High Pressure for 8 minutes.

4. After cooking, naturally release the pressure for 5 minutes, then quick release any remaining pressure.

5. Unlock and remove the lid. Carefully remove the eggs. Let cool before peeling.

6. Cut the eggs in half lengthwise. Remove the yolks, and set the whites aside. Put the yolks in a medium bowl.

7. Add the yogurt, mayonnaise, mustard, and hot sauce. Mash together until smooth. Season with salt and pepper.

8. Spoon or pipe the yolk mixture into the egg white halves.

9. Garnish with smoked paprika (if using). Refrigerate until ready to serve.

❖ **Ingredient Tip:** For best results, submerge the cooked eggs in a bowl of ice water for 5 minutes, then peel them as soon as they are cool enough to handle, since fully chilled eggs do not peel as easily.

Per Serving: Calories: 82; Fat: 5.5g; Protein: 7g; Carbohydrates: 1g; Fiber: 0g; Sugar: 0.5g; Sodium: 156mg

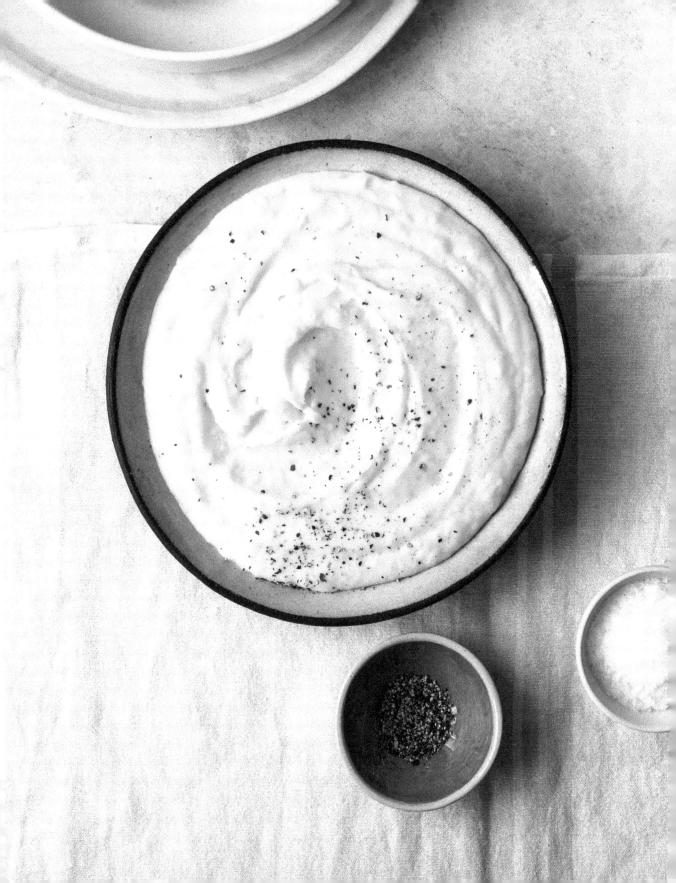

GARLIC-HERB MASHED POTATOES

Serves 6

Prep time: 5 minutes / **Pressure cook:** 8 minutes on High

Pressure release: Quick / **Total time:** 20 minutes

 5 OR FEWER INGREDIENTS   QUICK

Making this dish in the Instant Pot is a game changer. These creamy, fluffy mashed potatoes come together quickly, and there is no need to babysit a pot of boiling water. They have amazing garlic and herb flavor and are the perfect side dish for an everyday meal or a special holiday dinner. My favorite herbs are rosemary and thyme, but feel free to use whatever you have on hand.

---

2 cups water

2½ pounds russet potatoes, peeled and cut into 1-inch dice

3 garlic cloves, peeled

½ cup low-fat milk

⅓ cup 2 percent plain Greek yogurt

1 tablespoon chopped fresh herbs of choice, such as rosemary, thyme, or chives

Kosher salt

Freshly ground black pepper

1. In the inner pot, combine the water, potatoes, and garlic.

2. Lock the lid into place. Select Pressure Cook or Manual, and cook at High Pressure for 8 minutes.

3. After cooking, quick release the pressure.

4. Unlock and remove the lid. Drain the potatoes and garlic, and return to the pot.

5. Add the milk, yogurt, and herbs. Using a potato masher, mash the potatoes to your desired consistency. Season with salt and pepper.

❧ **Ingredient Tip:** Starchy potato varieties make for the creamiest, fluffiest mashed potatoes. I like russet and Idaho potatoes, but Yukon Gold would also work. If you are short on time, leave the skin on for extra flavor and texture.

Per Serving: Calories: 105; Fat: 0.5g; Protein: 4g; Carbohydrates: 22g; Fiber: 1.5g; Sugar: 2g; Sodium: 60mg

"SAUTÉED" MUSHROOMS

Serves 6

Prep time: 5 minutes / **Pressure cook:** 5 minutes on High; 7 minutes on Sauté
Pressure release: Quick / **Total time:** 25 minutes

5 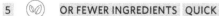 OR FEWER INGREDIENTS   QUICK

The best way to cook mushrooms is to take advantage of all the water they contain. Crowd them and add even more water, and they'll cook completely as they expel much of the water they contain. Once they're cooked, boil off the remaining water, and they'll brown perfectly, with a flavor so concentrated you won't believe it. I make a batch of these at least once a week to have on hand for all kinds of recipes. I highly recommend it.

---

1 pound white button or cremini mushrooms, washed and stems trimmed
1 tablespoon extra-virgin olive oil

½ teaspoon kosher salt
½ cup water

1. Cut medium mushrooms into quarters and large mushrooms into eighths.

2. Put the mushrooms, oil, salt, and water in the inner pot.

3. Lock the lid into place. Select Pressure Cook or Manual, and cook at High Pressure for 5 minutes.

4. After cooking, quick release the pressure.

5. Unlock and remove the lid. Select Sauté. Bring to a boil. Cook for about 5 minutes, or until all the water evaporates. The mushrooms will begin to sizzle in the remaining oil. Brown for 1 minute, then stir to brown the other sides for 1 minute more. Press Cancel to stop cooking. Serve warm.

♣ **Variation Tip:** Turn these into a delicious topping for steak or roasted chicken by adding 1 or 2 sliced shallots when the mushrooms have finished browning. Cook, stirring, for about 2 minutes, or until the shallots soften and start to brown. Pour in ¼ cup dry sherry, red wine, or dry white wine to deglaze the pan, scraping the browned bits from the bottom and letting most of the sherry evaporate. Season with salt and pepper.

Per Serving: Calories: 36; Fat: 2.5g; Protein: 1g; Carbohydrates: 3g; Fiber: 0g; Sugar: 2g; Sodium: 98mg

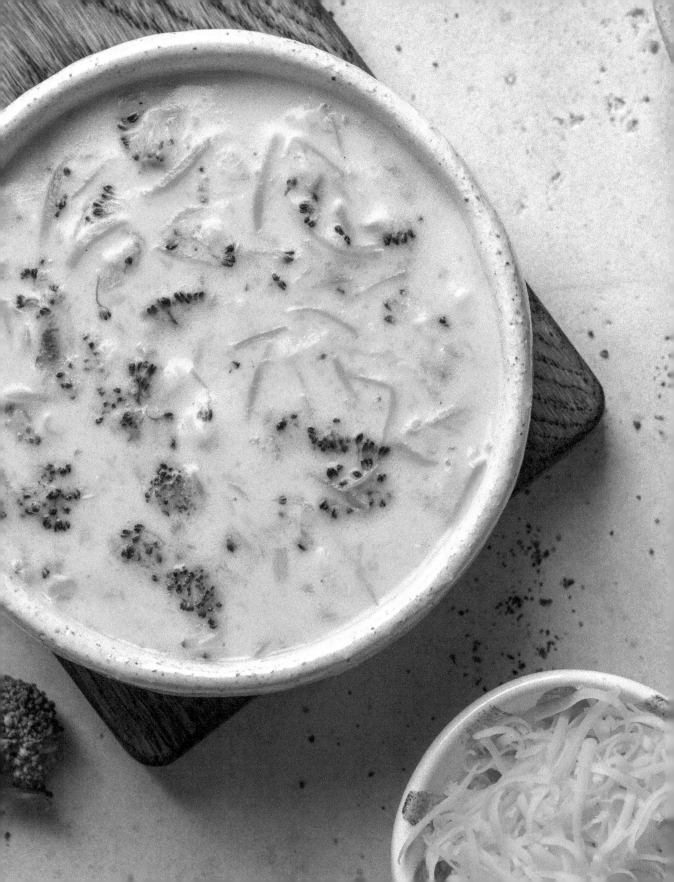

CHAPTER FOUR

Meatless Mains

BROCCOLI-CHEDDAR SOUP

Serves 6

Prep time: 10 minutes / **Pressure cook:** 5 minutes on Sauté; 3 minutes on High

Pressure release: Natural for 10 minutes, then Quick / **Total time:** 35 minutes

 ONE-POT MEAL

Broccoli and Cheddar cheese go so well together—think quiche, casserole, and, of course, soup. This soup is comforting, nourishing, and full of flavor. As a bonus, it is also gluten-free and really easy to pull together. To make it even easier, you can buy bags of prewashed, pre-chopped broccoli florets, either fresh or frozen.

1 tablespoon extra-virgin olive oil
1 medium yellow onion, chopped
2 garlic cloves, minced
3 cups Chicken Stock (page 137) or
   store-bought low-sodium chicken stock

1 pound fresh or frozen broccoli florets
   (about 3½ cups)
3 cups shredded Cheddar cheese
2 cups low-fat milk
Kosher salt
Freshly ground black pepper

1. Select Sauté, and pour the oil into the inner pot.

2. Once the oil is hot, add the onion and garlic. Sauté for about 2 minutes.

3. Add the stock. Using a wooden spoon, scrape up any browned bits stuck to the bottom of the pot.

4. Add the broccoli.

5. Lock the lid into place. Select Pressure Cook or Manual, and cook at High Pressure for 3 minutes (6 minutes if using frozen broccoli).

6. After cooking, naturally release the pressure for 10 minutes, then quick release any remaining pressure.

7. Unlock and remove the lid. Select Sauté. Stir in the cheese until melted and combined, followed by the milk. Let the soup come to a gentle simmer, then press Cancel. Season with salt and pepper. Serve immediately, or refrigerate in an airtight container for up to 4 days.

✿ **Substitution Tip:** To make this soup vegetarian, use vegetable stock instead of chicken stock.

Per Serving: Calories: 332; Fat: 22g; Protein: 22g; Carbohydrates: 12g; Fiber: 2g; Sugar: 6g; Sodium: 566mg

Lentil and Eggplant Stew

Serves 4

Prep time: 15 minutes / **Pressure cook:** 8 minutes on Sauté; 15 minutes on High

Pressure release: Natural for 15 minutes, then Quick / **Total time:** 1 hour 5 minutes

 ONE-POT MEAL WORTH THE WAIT

The most popular variety of eggplant looks like a large, pear-shaped egg—get it, "eggplant"?—and has a glossy, deep-purple skin and a cream-colored flesh that has a spongy consistency when raw. There are several varieties of eggplant available, all of which will taste great in this dish.

2 tablespoons extra-virgin olive oil
1 medium red onion, diced
4 thyme sprigs
4 garlic cloves, minced
1 teaspoon kosher salt
¼ teaspoon freshly ground black pepper
1 (1½-pound) eggplant, diced

1 pint cherry tomatoes
½ cup dry white wine
2 cups water
1 cup dried French green lentils, rinsed
  and drained
Crème fraîche, for serving (optional)

1. Select Sauté, and pour the oil into the inner pot.

2. Once the oil is hot, add the onion, and sauté for 3 minutes, or until the onion has softened.

3. Add the thyme, garlic, salt, and pepper. Sauté for 30 seconds, or until fragrant.

4. Add the eggplant and tomatoes. Sauté for 3 minutes, or until softened.

5. Add the wine, and deglaze: mix well, scrape up any brown bits, and reduce the wine for about 1 minute.

6. Add the water and lentils. Mix well.

7. Lock the lid into place. Select Pressure Cook or Manual, and cook at High Pressure for 15 minutes.

8. After cooking, naturally release the pressure for 15 minutes, then quick release any remaining pressure.

9. Unlock and remove the lid. Remove the thyme sprigs, add the lemon juice, and stir to mix.

10. Serve the stew warm, topped with crème fraîche (if using).

♻ **Ingredient Tip:** Diced eggplant cooks faster and fuses into the dish more than large chunks.

Per Serving: Calories: 320; Fat: 8g; Protein: 15g; Carbohydrates: 45g; Fiber: 20g; Sugar: 9g; Sodium: 300mg

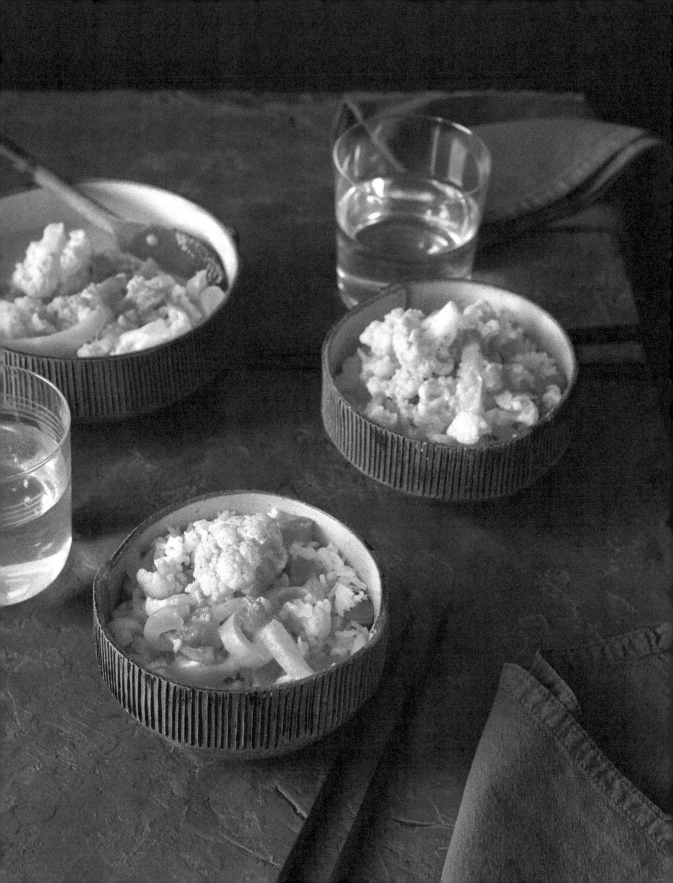

Coconut Red Curry Cauliflower

Serves 4 to 6

Prep time: 10 minutes / **Pressure cook:** 2 minutes on High

Pressure release: Quick / **Total time:** 20 minutes

 ONE-POT MEAL QUICK

Satisfy your takeout cravings with this easy curry. Serve it over rice, enjoy it on its own, or turn up the nutrient meter by stirring in your favorite greens at the end. This curry gets more flavorful the longer it sits, so leftovers make for great lunches. Of course, it's so delicious that it's hard not to eat it all the first time around!

---

1 (13½-ounce) can full-fat coconut milk

½ cup water

2 tablespoons red curry paste

1 teaspoon garlic powder

1 teaspoon kosher salt, plus more as needed

½ teaspoon ground ginger

½ teaspoon onion powder

¼ teaspoon chili powder or cayenne pepper

1 bell pepper, any color, cored and thinly sliced

1 small head cauliflower, cut into bite-size pieces (3 to 4 cups)

1 (14½-ounce) can diced tomatoes

Freshly ground black pepper

Cooked rice or other grain, for serving (optional)

1. In the inner pot, combine the coconut milk, water, red curry paste, garlic powder, salt, ginger, onion powder, and chili powder.

2. Add the bell pepper, cauliflower, and tomatoes with their juices. Stir.

3. Lock the lid into place. Select Pressure Cook or Manual, and cook at High Pressure for 2 minutes.

4. After cooking, quick release the pressure.

5. Unlock and remove the lid. Stir well. Season with salt and pepper.

6. Serve the curry with rice or another grain (if using).

❧ **Variation Tip:** Full-fat coconut milk helps make this curry rich and thick, but you can use the light, lower-fat version if you prefer.

Per Serving: Calories: 204; Fat: 17g; Protein: 4g; Carbohydrates: 11g; Fiber: 3.5g; Sugar: 4g; Sodium: 841mg

Quinoa and Corn Soup

Serves 4

Prep time: 10 minutes / **Pressure cook:** 4 minutes on High

Pressure release: Natural for 12 minutes, then Quick + Natural for 5 minutes, then Quick

Total time: 45 minutes

 ONE-POT MEAL

Adding quinoa to soup is an easy way to boost protein, but it can be hard to cook correctly. It tends to get gummy when cooked in soup, so I cook quinoa separately and add it at the end. This Southwestern-inspired soup makes for a great lunch.

1 cup quinoa, rinsed
5½ cups low-sodium vegetable stock, divided
1 small yellow onion, diced
2 garlic cloves, minced
1 small red bell pepper, cored and chopped
1 small green bell pepper, cored and chopped

1 small russet potato, peeled and cut into ½-inch dice
3 cups fresh or frozen corn
1 teaspoon ground cumin
1 teaspoon ground ancho chile
1 tablespoon freshly squeezed lime juice
Kosher salt

1. In the inner pot, combine the quinoa and 1½ cups of stock.

2. Lock the lid into place. Select Pressure Cook or Manual, and cook at High Pressure for 1 minute.

3. After cooking, naturally release the pressure for 12 minutes, then quick release any remaining pressure.

4. Unlock and remove the lid. Spoon the quinoa into a small bowl, and fluff with a fork.

5. In the inner pot, combine the remaining 4 cups of stock, the onion, garlic, red bell pepper, green bell pepper, potato, corn, cumin, and ground chile.

6. Lock the lid into place. Select Pressure Cook or Manual, and cook at High Pressure for 3 minutes.

7. After cooking, naturally release the pressure for 5 minutes, then quick release any remaining pressure.

8. Unlock and remove the lid. Add the quinoa to the soup.

9. Stir in the lime juice. Taste, and add salt if necessary. Ladle into soup bowls, and serve.

Per Serving: Calories: 327; Fat: 3.5g; Protein: 12g; Carbohydrates: 66g; Fiber: 8g; Sugar: 8.5g; Sodium: 272mg

BUTTERNUT SQUASH SOUP

Serves 6

Prep time: 5 minutes / **Pressure cook:** 3 minutes on Sauté; 13 minutes on High

Pressure release: Quick / **Total time:** 30 minutes

   ONE-POT MEAL   5 OR FEWER INGREDIENTS   QUICK

When squash is in season, it's an inexpensive and delicious ingredient in all kinds of recipes, but one of the easiest is soup. It does take some time to cut up the squash, but after that, you're less than 20 minutes away from a warming dish on a cold evening.

1 tablespoon extra-virgin olive oil

1 cup chopped yellow onion

Kosher salt

1 (2-pound) butternut squash, peeled, seeded, and cut into 1-inch chunks

6 cups low-sodium vegetable stock

½ teaspoon ground ginger

¼ teaspoon ground cayenne pepper

1. Preheat the Instant Pot by selecting Sauté.

2. Once hot, pour in the oil, and add the onion. Sprinkle with a pinch or two of salt. Cook, stirring, for about 3 minutes, or until the onion just begins to brown.

3. Add the squash, stock, ginger, and cayenne pepper. Stir to dissolve the spices.

4. Lock the lid into place. Select Pressure Cook or Manual, and cook at High Pressure for 13 minutes.

5. After cooking, quick release the pressure.

6. Unlock and remove the lid. Using an immersion or regular blender, puree the soup. Taste, and adjust the seasoning if needed. Ladle into bowls, and serve warm.

Per Serving: Calories: 108; Fat: 2.5g; Protein: 3g; Carbohydrates: 21g; Fiber: 4g; Sugar: 6g; Sodium: 193mg

→

Fennel and Leek Soup

Serves 4

Prep time: 5 minutes / **Pressure cook:** 2 minutes on Sauté; 7 minutes on High

Pressure release: Quick / **Total time:** 20 minutes

 ONE-POT MEAL QUICK

This is one of my favorite dishes to make when I crave a comforting bowl of soup yet want to keep it light and fresh. Leeks lend a distinct, subtle flavor, while the high starch content of the russet potato helps thicken the soup and make it delightfully creamy.

---

2 tablespoons extra-virgin olive oil

2 leeks, white and light green parts, washed and thinly sliced

2 garlic cloves, coarsely chopped

1 fennel bulb, fronds removed, cored, and thinly sliced

1 russet potato, peeled and diced

4 cups low-sodium vegetable stock

2 thyme sprigs

½ cup half-and-half

Kosher salt

Freshly ground black pepper

1. Select Sauté, and pour the oil into the inner pot.

2. Once the oil is hot, add the leeks and garlic. Sauté for 2 minutes.

3. Add the fennel, potato, stock, and thyme.

4. Lock the lid into place. Select Pressure Cook or Manual, and cook at High Pressure for 7 minutes.

5. After cooking, quick release the pressure.

6. Unlock and remove the lid. Remove and discard the thyme sprigs.

7. Using an immersion blender, traditional blender, or food processor, blend the soup until smooth.

8. Stir in the half-and-half. Season with salt and pepper.

♻ **Substitution Tip:** For a lighter soup, replace the half-and-half with milk. For a dairy-free version, you can substitute a nondairy milk alternative of your choice as long as it is unflavored and unsweetened.

Per Serving: Calories: 191; Fat: 20g; Protein: 4g; Carbohydrates: 23g; Fiber: 4g; Sugar: 7.5g; Sodium: 268mg

MUSHROOM-BARLEY RISOTTO

Serves 4

Prep time: 5 minutes / **Pressure cook:** 3 minutes on Sauté; 18 minutes on High

Pressure release: Natural for 10 minutes, then Quick / **Total time:** 45 minutes

 ONE-POT MEAL

Risotto can be a labor-intensive dish to cook, with the constant stirring and required supervision. Not with this barley risotto. Compared to traditional Arborio rice, barley provides a nutty flavor and chewy texture. Loaded with mushrooms, peas, and parmesan, this risotto is amazingly rich, creamy, and nutritious all around.

1 tablespoon extra-virgin olive oil
1 small yellow onion, diced
3 garlic cloves, minced
8 ounces cremini mushrooms, sliced
2 cups low-sodium vegetable stock
1 cup pearl barley, rinsed and drained

1 teaspoon dried thyme
¾ cup frozen peas, thawed
¼ cup grated parmesan cheese
Kosher salt
Freshly ground black pepper

1. Select Sauté, and pour the oil into the inner pot.

2. Once the oil is hot, add the onion, garlic, and mushrooms. Sauté for 3 minutes.

3. Add the stock, barley, and thyme.

4. Lock the lid into place. Select Pressure Cook or Manual, and cook at High Pressure for 18 minutes.

5. After cooking, naturally release the pressure for 10 minutes, then quick release any remaining pressure.

6. Unlock and remove the lid. Stir in the peas and cheese for about 1 minute, or until heated through. Season with salt and pepper.

♣ **Ingredient Tip:** To add more flavor to this dish, use a mixture of fresh or dried mushrooms, such as porcini, shiitake, portabella, or oyster.

Per Serving: Calories: 279; Fat: 5.5g; Protein: 10g; Carbohydrates: 50g; Fiber: 10g; Sugar: 4g; Sodium: 257mg

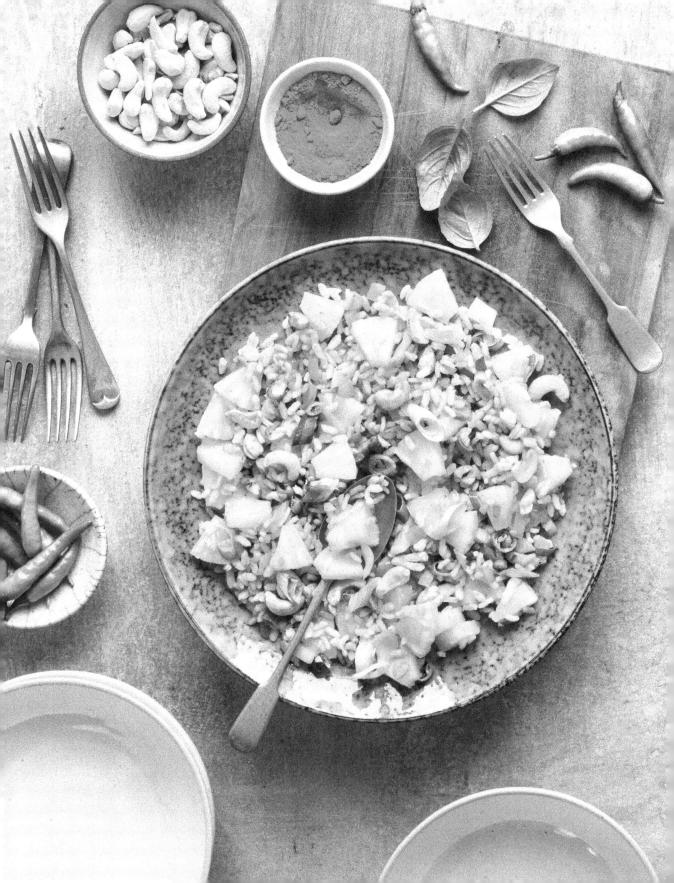

Thai-Inspired Pineapple Fried Rice

Serves 4

Prep time: 10 minutes, plus 15 minutes to cool
Pressure cook: 5 minutes on Sauté; 3 minutes on High
Pressure release: Natural for 3 minutes, then Quick / **Total time:** 45 minutes

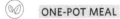 ONE-POT MEAL

The mix of sweet pineapple and savory cashews in this fried rice is irresistible. Leftover rice is ideal—that extra time in the refrigerator allows it to dry out a bit. Pair with the Coconut Red Curry Cauliflower (page 55) for a perfect meal.

---

1 tablespoon vegetable oil
¼ cup whole cashews
¼ cup finely chopped yellow onion
¼ cup finely chopped scallions, white parts only
2 green Thai chiles, finely chopped
1 cup canned pineapple chunks
¼ cup coarsely chopped fresh basil
  leaves, divided

2 teaspoons reduced-sodium soy sauce
1 teaspoon kosher salt
½ teaspoon curry powder
¼ teaspoon ground turmeric
1 cup steamed short-grain white rice
¼ cup water

1. Select Sauté, and pour the oil into the inner pot.

2. Once the oil is hot, add the cashews, and sauté for 1 minute.

3. Add the onion, scallions, and chiles. Sauté for 3 to 4 minutes, or until the onion is translucent.

4. Mix in the pineapple, 2 tablespoons of basil, the soy sauce, salt, curry powder, and turmeric.

5. Add the rice and water. Mix again.

6. Lock the lid into place. Select Pressure Cook or Manual, and cook at High Pressure for 3 minutes.

7. After cooking, naturally release the pressure for 3 minutes, then quick release any remaining pressure.

8. Unlock and remove the lid. Let the rice cool for 15 minutes. Using a fork, fluff the rice. Serve warm.

❖ **Substitution Tip:** To make this gluten-free, use tamari instead of soy sauce (make sure the label says gluten-free).

Per Serving: Calories: 179; Fat: 6.5g; Protein: 3g; Carbohydrates: 27g; Fiber: 1.5g; Sugar: 10g; Sodium: 379mg

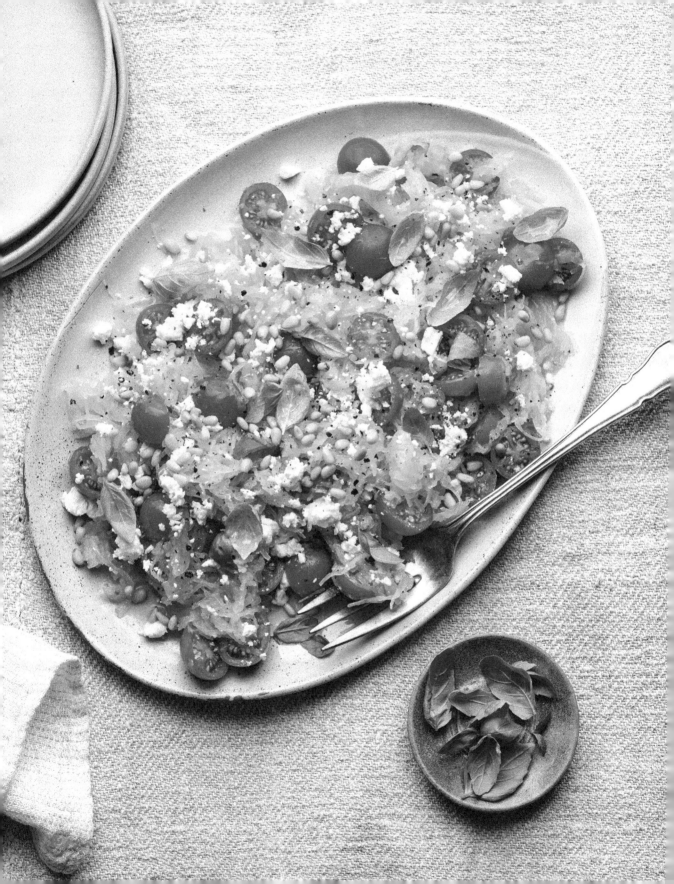

Spaghetti Squash with Cherry Tomatoes, Basil, and Feta

Serves 4

Prep time: 15 minutes / **Pressure cook:** 10 minutes on High

Pressure release: Quick / **Total time:** 35 minutes

Part of the winter squash family, spaghetti squash is typically large, yellow skinned, and oblong with a flesh that pulls away in strands resembling spaghetti when cooked. It is neutral in flavor, has a tender and chewy texture, and is often used as a swap-in for pasta or grains. It is low in calories but nutrient dense.

1½ cups water

1 (3- to 3½-pound) spaghetti squash, halved and seeded

2 pints cherry tomatoes, halved

½ cup crumbled feta cheese

2 tablespoons extra-virgin olive oil

2 tablespoons freshly squeezed lemon juice

½ teaspoon kosher salt

¼ teaspoon freshly ground black pepper

$\frac{1}{3}$ cup pine nuts, toasted

¼ cup fresh basil leaves (optional)

1. Pour the water into the Instant Pot.

2. Add the squash, skin-side down and angled so as not to completely cover one half with the other half.

3. Lock the lid into place. Select Pressure Cook or Manual, and cook at High Pressure for 10 minutes.

4. After cooking, quick release the pressure.

5. Unlock and remove the lid. Carefully transfer the squash to a cutting board. Using a fork, scrape the flesh out of the squash halves; it should come out easily and look similar to spaghetti.

6. In a large bowl, toss together the tomatoes, cheese, oil, lemon juice, salt, and pepper.

7. Add the squash strands, and toss.

8. Garnish with the pine nuts and basil (if using), and serve warm.

♻ **Ingredient Tip:** Sometimes spaghetti squash can be difficult to cut in half. To make it easier, simply microwave the squash in 30-second intervals until you are able to cut it in half.

Per Serving: Calories: 294; Fat: 20g; Protein: 7g; Carbohydrates: 27g; Fiber: 6g; Sugar: 12g; Sodium: 364mg

CARIBBEAN-STYLE BEANS AND RICE

Serves 4

Prep time: 15 minutes, plus 6 hours to soak

Pressure cook: 13 minutes on High; 7 minutes on Sauté

Pressure release: Natural + Natural for 5 minutes, then Quick / **Total time:** 6 hours 50 minutes

 WORTH THE WAIT

Caribbean cuisine is known for its use of spices and coconut. A traditional recipe for Caribbean beans and rice calls for a very hot Scotch bonnet pepper. My take uses the much milder jalapeño pepper. The coconut milk not only balances the heat but also makes the rice rich and creamy.

⅓ cup dried kidney beans

2 cups water

1 teaspoon vegetable oil

1 medium yellow onion, diced

2 garlic cloves, minced

2 teaspoons seeded and finely chopped
  jalapeño pepper

1 tomato, finely chopped

1 teaspoon dried thyme

1 teaspoon kosher salt

1 cup full-fat coconut milk

⅔ cup basmati rice, rinsed and drained

1. In a large bowl, cover the kidney beans with 2 to 3 inches of cold water. Soak at room temperature for 6 hours. Drain and rinse.

2. Pour the water into the inner pot, and add the beans.

3. Lock the lid into place. Select Pressure Cook or Manual, and cook at High Pressure for 10 minutes.

4. After cooking, naturally release the pressure.

5. Unlock and remove the lid. Drain the beans, reserving and setting aside ½ cup of the bean water. Set the beans aside in a medium bowl. Wipe the inner pot dry.

6. Select Sauté, and pour the oil into the inner pot.

7. Once the oil is hot, add the onion, garlic, and jalapeño. Sauté for about 5 minutes, or until the onion is translucent.

8. Stir in the tomato, thyme, and salt. Cook for 2 minutes.

9. Pour the reserved bean water into the inner pot. Stir in the coconut milk and rice.

10. Lock the lid into place. Select Pressure Cook or Manual, and cook at High Pressure for 3 minutes.

11. After cooking, naturally release the pressure for 5 minutes, then quick release any remaining pressure.

12. Unlock and remove the lid. Let the rice cool for 5 minutes, then fluff with a fork and serve with the beans.

♻ **Variation Tip:** Double the recipe by doubling all the ingredients, including the water, but not the cooking time. If using a mini, make sure you don't fill the pot more than two-thirds full; otherwise, it will overflow.

Per Serving: Calories: 300; Fat: 13g; Protein: 8g; Carbohydrates: 38g; Fiber: 5g; Sugar: 1g; Sodium: 291mg

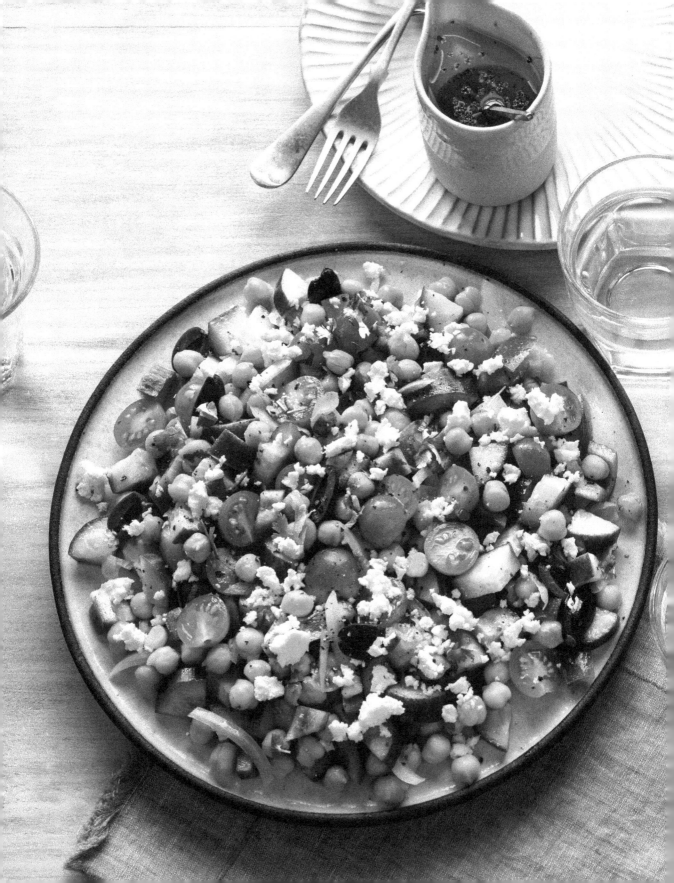

CHICKPEA GREEK SALAD

Serves 6

Prep time: 10 minutes, plus 6 hours to soak / **Pressure cook:** 15 minutes on High

Pressure release: Natural / **Total time:** 6 hours 35 minutes

 WORTH THE WAIT

Healthy, light, and refreshing, this Mediterranean-style chickpea salad is tossed with a red-wine vinegar dressing. Cook a large batch of chickpeas over the weekend, and make this your go-to weekday meal. Skip the feta to make this salad vegan.

---

1 cup dried chickpeas

3 cups water

2 tablespoons extra-virgin olive oil

1 tablespoon red-wine vinegar

1 teaspoon kosher salt

½ teaspoon freshly ground black pepper

½ cup finely chopped onion

10 cherry tomatoes, halved

10 pitted black olives, halved

1 cucumber, cut into ½-inch dice

¼ cup chopped green bell pepper

2 tablespoons finely chopped fresh cilantro

1 ounce feta cheese, crumbled

1. In a large bowl, cover the chickpeas with 2 to 3 inches of cold water. Soak at room temperature for 6 to 8 hours or overnight. Drain and rinse.

2. Pour the water into the inner pot, and add the chickpeas.

3. Lock the lid into place. Select Pressure Cook or Manual, and cook at High Pressure for 15 minutes.

4. After cooking, naturally release the pressure.

5. Unlock and remove the lid. Drain the chickpeas. Let cool for about 5 minutes.

6. To make the dressing, in a small jar or bowl, combine the oil, vinegar, salt, and pepper. Seal and shake, or whisk thoroughly.

7. In a large bowl, combine the chickpeas, onion, tomatoes, olives, cucumber, bell pepper, and cilantro.

8. Add the dressing, and toss.

9. Top with the cheese, and serve.

✿ **Variation Tip:** You can make this salad with kidney beans or navy beans. You won't need to adjust the pressure or cook time for either swap.

Per Serving: Calories: 203; Fat: 9g; Protein: 8g; Carbohydrates: 24g; Fiber: 7.5g; Sugar: 5.5g; Sodium: 344mg

SOUTHWESTERN TOFU SCRAMBLE

Serves 4

Prep time: 5 minutes / **Pressure cook:** 3 minutes on Sauté; 3 minutes on High
Pressure release: Quick / **Total time:** 20 minutes

 ONE-POT MEAL QUICK

Tofu is one of my favorite ingredients to cook with. It's incredibly versatile and has a mild taste, which makes it perfect for soaking up flavor in a variety of dishes. This scrumptious vegan dish is loaded with tasty spices and cooks quickly for a filling, protein-packed breakfast, lunch, or dinner.

---

1 tablespoon extra-virgin olive oil
1 medium yellow onion, diced
2 garlic cloves, minced
1 red bell pepper, cored and diced
1 (16-ounce) block firm tofu, drained and crumbled
1 bunch kale, stemmed and chopped
1 tablespoon chili powder
1 teaspoon ground cumin
½ teaspoon ground cayenne pepper (optional)
Kosher salt
Freshly ground black pepper

1. Select Sauté, and pour the oil into the inner pot.

2. Once the oil is hot, add the onion, garlic, and bell pepper. Sauté for 3 minutes.

3. Add the tofu, kale, chili powder, cumin, and cayenne pepper (if using).

4. Lock the lid into place. Select Pressure Cook or Manual, and cook at High Pressure for 3 minutes.

5. After cooking, quick release the pressure.

6. Unlock and remove the lid. Season the scramble with salt and pepper.

❧ **Substitution Tip:** Other hearty greens such as chard (Swiss or rainbow), escarole, or collard greens can be used in place of the kale.

Per Serving: Calories: 183; Fat: 9g; Protein: 14g; Carbohydrates: 14g; Fiber: 4.5g; Sugar: 4.5g; Sodium: 130mg

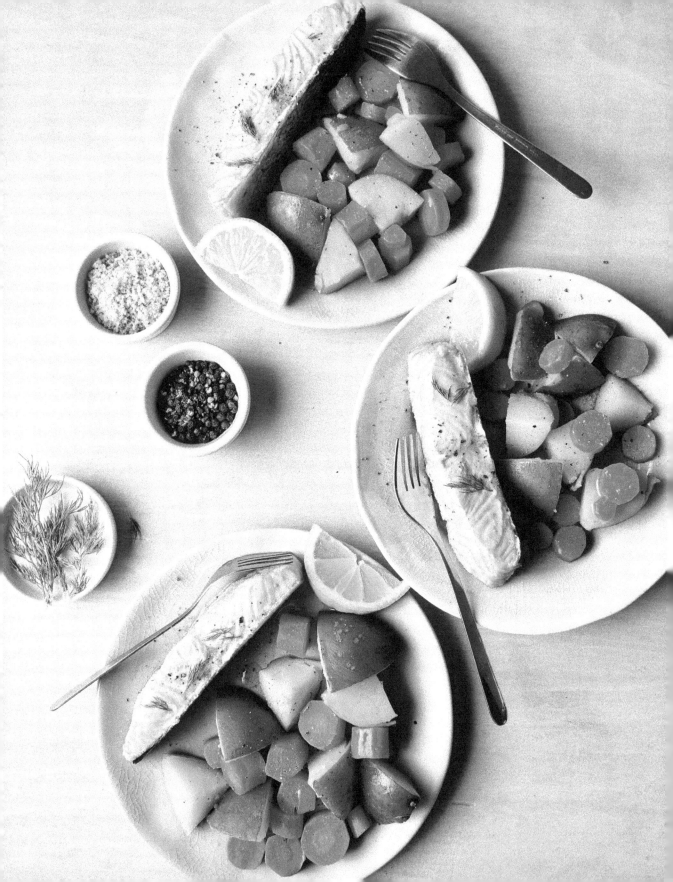

CHAPTER FIVE

Fish and Shellfish

SALMON AND VEGETABLES WITH LEMON-BUTTER SAUCE

Serves 5
Prep time: 10 minutes / **Pressure cook:** 5 minutes on High
Pressure release: Natural for 10 minutes, then Quick / **Total time:** 35 minutes

 ONE-POT MEAL

Don't you love when a showstopping dish is actually one of the simplest to make? This recipe is the perfect example. You don't even have to plan ahead; just grab salmon fillets out of the freezer, and cook them right along with red potatoes and carrots. The butter sauce coats everything and makes for a flavorful, healthy meal.

1 cup low-sodium vegetable stock
2 pounds medium red potatoes, cut into 1-inch chunks
4 medium carrots, chopped into 1-inch-thick pieces
5 (4-ounce) frozen skin-on salmon fillets

4 tablespoons (½ stick) unsalted butter, melted
1 teaspoon kosher salt
½ teaspoon garlic powder
Juice of 2 lemons
Freshly ground black pepper, for garnish
Fresh chopped dill, for garnish (optional)

1. Pour the stock into the inner pot, and add the potatoes and carrots.

2. Place the fillets, skin-side down, on top of the vegetables.

3. Pour the melted butter over the fillets. Sprinkle with the salt and garlic powder.

4. Lock the lid into place. Select Pressure Cook or Manual, and cook at High Pressure for 5 minutes.

5. After cooking, naturally release the pressure for 10 minutes, then quick release any remaining pressure.

6. Unlock and remove the lid. Add the lemon juice.

7. Serve the salmon and vegetables immediately, garnished with pepper and dill (if using).

✿ **Ingredient Tip:** If your salmon fillets are larger than 4 ounces, you might be able to fit only four in the pot at a time. Also, be sure to cut your potatoes and vegetables fairly small so they cook all the way through during the short cooking time.

Per Serving: Calories: 396; Fat: 17g; Protein: 27g; Carbohydrates: 35g; Fiber: 4.5g; Sugar: 5.5g; Sodium: 369mg

Mussels with Red Pepper-Garlic Sauce

Serves 4

Prep time: 15 minutes / **Pressure cook:** 1 minute on Sauté; 1 minute on High

Pressure release: Quick / **Total time:** 25 minutes

 ONE-POT MEAL QUICK

There's something comforting about digging into a big bowl of steamed mussels with a savory broth. In this recipe, the roasted red pepper gives a hint of sweetness to the broth, which complements the mussels perfectly. It's also fabulous for sopping up with plenty of crusty bread. It's definitely one of those dishes that will impress anyone you serve it to—despite how easy it is to make!

---

3 pounds mussels

1 tablespoon extra-virgin olive oil

4 garlic cloves, minced

1 large roasted red bell pepper, minced
  or pureed

¾ cup fish stock, clam juice, or water

½ cup dry white wine

⅛ teaspoon red pepper flakes

2 tablespoons heavy cream

3 tablespoons coarsely chopped fresh parsley

1. Scrub the mussels, and debeard if necessary (some fish counters sell debearded mussels).

2. Select Sauté, and pour the oil into the inner pot.

3. Once the oil is hot, add the garlic, and sauté for about 1 minute, or until fragrant.

4. Add the roasted red pepper, fish stock, wine, and red pepper flakes. Stir to combine.

5. Add the mussels.

6. Lock the lid into place. Select Pressure Cook or Manual, and cook at High Pressure for 1 minute.

7. After cooking, quick release the pressure.

8. Unlock and remove the lid. Check the mussels; if they have not opened, replace the lid but don't lock it into place. Let the mussels steam for 1 minute, or until they've opened. (Discard any that do not open.)

9. Stir in the cream and parsley.

10. Serve the mussels with the cooking liquid.

Per Serving: Calories: 394; Fat: 14g; Protein: 42g; Carbohydrates: 16g; Fiber: 0.5g; Sugar: 1.5g; Sodium: 1,046mg

STEAMED CLAMS

Serves 4

Prep time: 10 minutes / **Pressure cook:** 4 minutes on High

Pressure release: Natural for 15 minutes, then Quick / **Total time:** 40 minutes

 ONE-POT MEAL

Steamed clams are an easy, delicious dinner if you're in the mood for a pot of seafood. Clam shells can be fairly sandy, so be sure to scrub them well with a plastic brush prior to cooking. If any clam shells do not open after cooking, place the lid back on top askew, turn on the sauté function, and simmer for a few minutes until they open. If there are any remaining that do not open, discard them before serving.

---

4 pounds littleneck clams, washed and scrubbed

1 cup low-sodium vegetable stock

1 cup dry white wine

¼ cup chopped fresh basil leaves

2 tablespoons freshly squeezed lemon juice

1 tablespoon extra-virgin olive oil

Crusty bread, for serving

1. In the inner pot, combine the clams, stock, wine, basil, lemon juice, and oil.

2. Lock the lid into place. Select Pressure Cook or Manual, and cook at High Pressure for 4 minutes.

3. After cooking, naturally release the pressure for 15 minutes, then quick release any remaining pressure.

4. Unlock and remove the lid. If some clams are still closed, press the sauté button, and simmer for 1 to 2 minutes. Press Cancel to stop cooking. Transfer to a serving dish. (Discard any that do not open.)

5. Serve the clams warm with crusty bread.

❖ **Variation Tip:** If you cannot find littleneck clams or simply prefer a different type, any clams will work well in this recipe.

Per Serving: Calories: 340; Fat: 4g; Protein: 58g; Carbohydrates: 13g; Fiber: 1g; Sugar: 1g; Sodium: 320mg

Peel-and-Eat Shrimp with Two Sauces

Serves 4

Prep time: 15 minutes / **Pressure cook:** 1 minute on Low

Pressure release: Quick / **Total time:** 25 minutes

 QUICK

I know what you're thinking—shrimp in an Instant Pot? Won't they be overcooked? That's exactly what I thought at first until I started experimenting with frozen shell-on shrimp. Turns out that if they go in frozen, protected by their shells, shrimp turn out perfect. Make a couple of classic sauces while the shrimp cook, and you have a great appetizer for any occasion.

FOR THE SHRIMP

1 cup water

2 pounds frozen jumbo ($^{16}/_{25}$ count) shell-on shrimp

FOR THE COCKTAIL SAUCE

½ cup ketchup

1 tablespoon prepared horseradish

1 tablespoon freshly squeezed lemon juice

½ teaspoon Worcestershire sauce

Dash hot sauce, such as Tabasco

$^1/_8$ teaspoon celery salt

FOR THE REMOULADE

¼ cup plain low-fat yogurt

¼ cup mayonnaise

2 tablespoons ketchup

2 tablespoons Creole mustard or other grainy mustard

2 teaspoons prepared horseradish

½ teaspoon Worcestershire sauce

2 scallions, green and white parts, coarsely chopped

2 tablespoons coarsely chopped fresh parsley leaves

TO MAKE THE SHRIMP

1. Pour the water into the Instant Pot.

2. Arrange the frozen shrimp in a single layer (as much as possible) in a steamer basket, and place it inside.

3. Lock the lid into place. Select Steam, and cook at Low Pressure for 1 minute.

4. Meanwhile, fill a large bowl about halfway with cold water. Add several handfuls of ice cubes.

5. After cooking, quick release the pressure.

6. Unlock and remove the lid. Take the steam basket out. Transfer the shrimp to the ice bath.

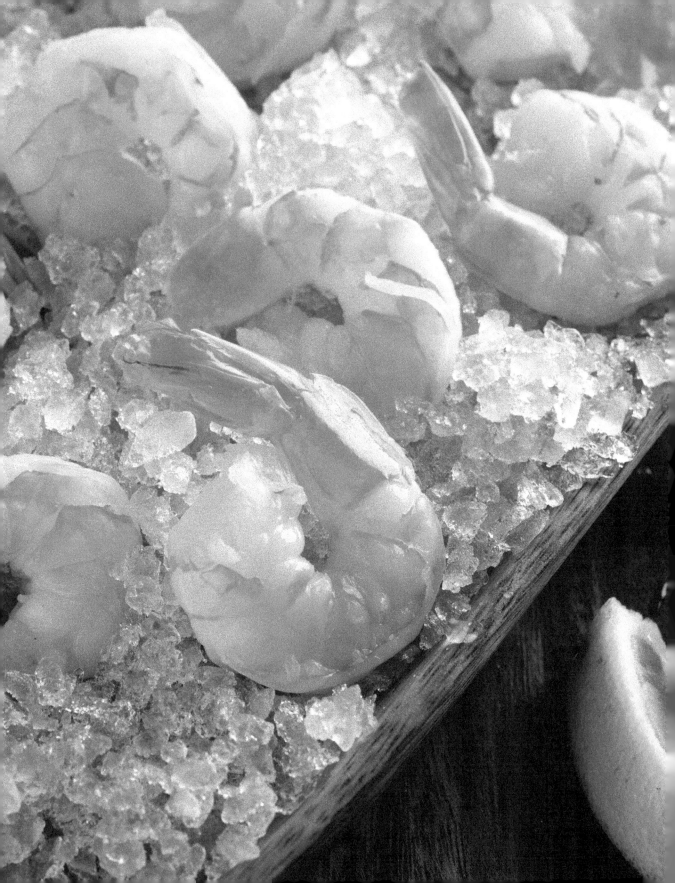

TO MAKE THE COCKTAIL SAUCE

7. In a small bowl, mix together the ketchup, horseradish, lemon juice, Worcestershire sauce, hot sauce, and celery salt. Whisk until smooth. Adjust the seasoning if necessary.

TO MAKE THE REMOULADE

8. Put the yogurt, mayonnaise, ketchup, mustard, horseradish, Worcestershire sauce, scallions, and parsley in a small food processor. Process until mostly smooth, scraping down the sides of the bowl as necessary. (If you don't have a food processor, whisk together the yogurt, mayonnaise, ketchup, mustard, horseradish, and Worcestershire sauce. Mince the scallions and parsley, and stir into the sauce.)

9. Arrange the shrimp on a large platter with the dipping sauces in ramekins. Provide a bowl for the shells—and lots of napkins.

♻ **Ingredient Tip:** If your shrimp are smaller, follow the same procedure, but cook for 0 minutes at Low Pressure. The smallest shrimp I recommend for this recipe are 26/30 count.

Per Serving: Calories: 337; Fat: 12g; Protein: 40g; Carbohydrates: 16g; Fiber: 0.5g; Sugar: 12g; Sodium: 933mg

→

MONKFISH WITH KALE AND WHITE BEANS

Serves 4

Prep time: 15 minutes / **Pressure cook:** 3 minutes on Sauté; 5 minutes on High

Pressure release: Natural for 10 minutes, then Quick / **Total time:** 40 minutes

 ONE-POT MEAL

Monkfish has a mild, slightly sweet taste and is dense, firm, and boneless, similar to lobster tail. Its firm texture means it will not fall apart when cooked, so it typically holds up very well in the Instant Pot.

---

2 tablespoons extra-virgin olive oil
1 small yellow onion, diced
1 tablespoon minced fresh rosemary leaves
2 garlic cloves, minced
¾ teaspoon kosher salt
¼ teaspoon red pepper flakes
½ cup dry white wine

½ cup low-sodium vegetable stock
1 bunch kale, stemmed and chopped
1 (15-ounce) can cannellini beans, rinsed
  and drained
1 pound monkfish fillets
Juice of ½ lemon

1. Select Sauté on the Instant Pot, allow it to heat up, then pour in the oil.

2. Add the onion, and sauté for 2 minutes, or until softened.

3. Add the rosemary, garlic, salt, and red pepper flakes. Sauté for 30 seconds, or until fragrant.

4. Add the wine, and deglaze: mix well, and scrape up any brown bits on the bottom of the pot.

5. Add the stock, kale, and beans. Mix well.

6. Nestle the monkfish fillets into the pot.

7. Lock the lid into place. Select Pressure Cook or Manual, and cook at High Pressure for 5 minutes.

8. After cooking, naturally release the pressure for 10 minutes, then quick release any remaining pressure.

9. Unlock and remove the lid, then mix well. The fish should be cooked through and opaque. If it is not quite cooked through, select Sauté, place the lid askew over the pot, and simmer until finished. Press Cancel to stop cooking.

10. Add the lemon juice, and mix well. Serve.

✿ **Ingredient Tip:** For faster prep, use pre-packaged chopped kale or baby kale instead.

Per Serving: Calories: 330; Fat: 9g; Protein: 27g; Carbohydrates: 30g; Fiber: 8g; Sugar: 3g; Sodium: 270mg

Coconut Fish Curry

Serves 6

Prep time: 10 minutes / **Pressure cook:** 4 minutes on Sauté; 4 minutes on High
Pressure release: Natural for 10 minutes, then Quick / **Total time:** 35 minutes

 ONE-POT MEAL

This recipe is inspired by a fish curry I had while on vacation on the island of Maui in Hawaii. I make my version with firm white fish and canned coconut milk, and the fish comes out perfectly cooked, surrounded by flavorful broth and lots of crunchy vegetables. I like to serve this dish Hawaiian-style in a shallow bowl with a scoop of basmati rice on the side.

2 tablespoons extra-virgin olive oil
1 small yellow onion, sliced
1½ pounds mahi mahi fillets (about 4 fillets),
    cut into 2-inch dice
1 tablespoon green curry paste
1 (13½-ounce) can full-fat coconut milk

2 tablespoons reduced-sodium soy sauce
1 tablespoon brown sugar
½ teaspoon ground ginger
2 red bell peppers, cored and sliced
Juice of 1 lime

1. Select Sauté, and pour the oil into the inner pot.

2. Once the oil is hot, add the onion, fillets, and green curry paste. Sauté, stirring occasionally, for about 4 minutes, or until the fillets have browned on all sides.

3. Add the coconut milk, soy sauce, sugar, and ginger. Using a wooden spoon, scrape up any browned bits stuck to the bottom of the pot.

4. Add the bell peppers, and stir to combine.

5. Lock the lid into place. Select Pressure Cook or Manual, and cook at High Pressure for 4 minutes.

6. After cooking, naturally release the pressure for 10 minutes, then quick release any remaining pressure.

7. Unlock and remove the lid. Stir in the lime juice.

8. Serve the curry immediately, refrigerate in an airtight container for up to 4 days, or freeze for up to 2 months.

❖ **Substitution Tip:** To make this gluten-free, use tamari in place of the soy sauce.

Per Serving: Calories: 293; Fat: 19g; Protein: 23g; Carbohydrates: 9g; Fiber: 1.5g; Sugar: 4.5g; Sodium: 386mg

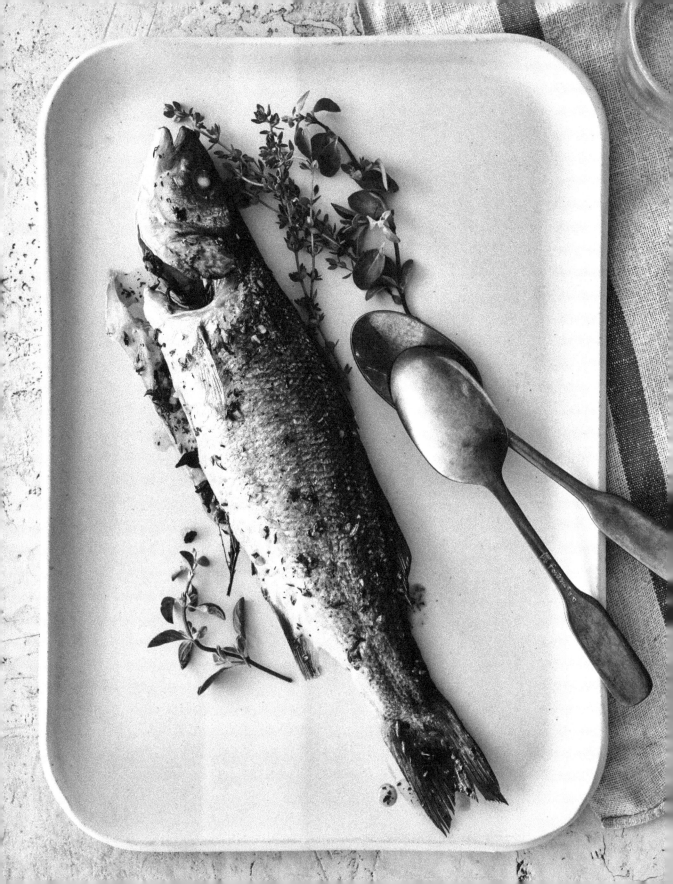

WHOLE BRANZINO

Serves 4

Prep time: 5 minutes / **Pressure cook:** 7 minutes on High

Pressure release: Quick / **Total time:** 20 minutes

5 OR FEWER INGREDIENTS QUICK

Branzino has been called European bass and is very popular in Mediterranean cuisine. Cooking and serving a whole fish doesn't have to be reserved for restaurant meals! This simple, tasty, and healthy recipe can easily be made any day of the week. To round out the meal, serve it with Garlicky Lemon Broccoli (page 41) and Cilantro-Lime Rice (page 44).

---

2 whole branzino, cleaned and scaled
1 teaspoon kosher salt
½ teaspoon freshly ground black pepper
1 cup water

Nonstick cooking spray, for coating the
  steam rack
1 lemon, thinly sliced, divided

1. Season the inside of the branzino with the salt and pepper.

2. Pour the water into the Instant Pot.

3. Coat a steam rack with cooking spray, and place inside the pot, handles extending up.

4. Place the branzino on the prepared steam rack.

5. Place the lemon slices on top of the fish.

6. Lock the lid into place. Select Pressure Cook or Manual, and cook at High Pressure for 7 minutes.

7. After cooking, quick release the pressure.

8. Unlock and remove the lid. Carefully remove the steam rack with the branzino.

9. Place the branzino on a serving platter. Remove the fillets; they should easily separate and pull away from the bones. Serve immediately.

♻ **Variation Tip:** Any whole fish or large side of fish or fillet that can fit in your Instant Pot would work well with this recipe. Just be sure the fish you choose has been cleaned and scaled.

Per Serving: Calories: 245; Fat: 8.5g; Protein: 42g; Carbohydrates: 0g; Fiber: 0g; Sugar: 0g; Sodium: 434mg

COD AND POTATO STEW

Serves 4

Prep time: 5 minutes / **Pressure cook:** 9 minutes on Sauté; 10 minutes on High

Pressure release: Quick / **Total time:** 35 minutes

 ONE-POT MEAL

Potatoes and fish are always a complementary combination, and the addition of shallots and fennel permeates the stew with their aromatic flavors. Instead of cod, you can use another fish as long as it is mildly flavored and has a firm texture that holds up to stewing without falling apart. Sea bass, haddock, and halibut are all good options.

2 tablespoons extra-virgin olive oil

1 fennel bulb, fronds removed and diced

2 shallots, diced

2 garlic cloves, minced

8 ounces baby Yukon Gold or red potatoes, skin-on and halved

2 cups low-sodium fish stock or Chicken Stock (page 137)

½ cup dry white wine

1½ pounds cod, cut into 2-inch pieces

¼ cup half-and-half

2 tablespoons chopped fresh dill

Kosher salt

Freshly ground black pepper

1. Select Sauté, and pour the oil into the inner pot.

2. Once the oil is hot, add the fennel, shallots, and garlic. Sauté for 4 minutes.

3. Add the potatoes, stock, and wine.

4. Lock the lid into place. Select Pressure Cook or Manual, and cook at High Pressure for 10 minutes.

5. After cooking, quick release the pressure.

6. Select Sauté, and bring the stew to a simmer. Then add the cod, and simmer for about 5 minutes, or until just cooked through. Press Cancel to stop cooking.

7. Stir in the half-and-half and dill. Season the stew with salt and pepper.

♻ **Variation Tip:** For a thicker stew, remove 1 cup of the cooked vegetables and 1 cup of the broth, and puree in a blender until smooth. Return to the pot, and stir before adding the cod.

Per Serving: Calories: 340; Fat: 10g; Protein: 36g; Carbohydrates: 21g; Fiber: 3.5g; Sugar: 5g; Sodium: 405mg

NEW ENGLAND CLAM CHOWDER

Serves 4

Prep time: 5 minutes / **Pressure cook:** 11 minutes on Sauté; 7 minutes on High

Pressure release: Quick / **Total time:** 35 minutes

 ONE-POT MEAL

This New England–style chowder is made with milk instead of heavy cream, reducing the calories significantly. Bacon is used, but you can use turkey bacon if you prefer.

---

4 bacon slices, diced

1 medium yellow onion, diced

2 garlic cloves, minced

2 celery stalks, diced

1 large carrot, diced

1 pound Yukon Gold potatoes, peeled and diced

2 cups clam juice

2 (6½-ounce) cans chopped clams, strained and juice reserved

1 bay leaf

½ teaspoon dried thyme

2 cups low-fat milk

2 tablespoons cornstarch

Kosher salt

Freshly ground black pepper

Fresh chopped chives, for garnish

1. Line a plate with paper towels. Select Sauté, put the bacon in the Instant Pot, and cook for about 5 minutes, or until crisp. Transfer the bacon to the prepared plate. Retain about 1 tablespoon of bacon fat in the pot.

2. Add the onion and garlic. Cook for 2 minutes, or until the onion is soft.

3. Add the celery, carrot, potatoes, clam juice, reserved liquid from the clams, bay leaf, and thyme. Stir to combine.

4. Lock the lid into place. Select Pressure Cook or Manual, and cook at High Pressure for 7 minutes.

5. After cooking, quick release the pressure.

6. In a bowl, whisk together the milk and cornstarch. Select Sauté, and bring the chowder to a simmer.

7. Once the chowder is simmering, stir in the cornstarch mixture, clams, and bacon. Simmer for 3 minutes. Press Cancel to stop cooking. Season with salt and pepper.

8. Garnish with chives before serving.

Per Serving: Calories: 389; Fat: 13g; Protein: 27g; Carbohydrates: 40g; Fiber: 3.5g; Sugar: 9.5g; Sodium: 965mg

SHRIMP SCAMPI PASTA

Serves 6

Prep time: 5 minutes / **Pressure cook:** 8 minutes on Sauté; 3 minutes on High

Pressure release: Quick / **Total time:** 25 minutes

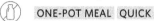 ONE-POT MEAL QUICK

My husband's all-time favorite, this is the type of recipe to keep up your sleeve whenever you need a scrumptious meal that is as good for a weeknight dinner as it is for entertaining. I hope you love it as much as my family and I do!

---

2 tablespoons extra-virgin olive oil	¼ cup dry white wine
2 shallots, diced	3 cups low-sodium chicken stock
3 garlic cloves, minced	12 ounces rotini
1 pound large shrimp, peeled and deveined	1 teaspoon grated lemon zest
½ teaspoon kosher salt, plus more as needed	2 tablespoons freshly squeezed lemon juice
¼ teaspoon freshly ground black pepper, plus more as needed	¼ teaspoon red pepper flakes
	2 tablespoons chopped fresh parsley

1. Select Sauté, and pour the oil into the inner pot.

2. Once the oil is hot, add the shallots and garlic. Sauté for 2 minutes.

3. Add the shrimp. Season with the salt and pepper. Cook for 1 to 2 minutes per side, or until the shrimp turn pink. Using a slotted spoon, remove the shrimp to a plate.

4. Add the wine to the pot, and simmer for 2 minutes, or until reduced by about half.

5. Add the chicken stock and rotini.

6. Lock the lid into place. Select Pressure Cook or Manual, and cook at High Pressure for 3 minutes.

7. After cooking, quick release the pressure.

8. Stir in the cooked shrimp, lemon zest, lemon juice, and red pepper flakes. Season with salt and pepper.

9. Garnish with the parsley before serving.

✣ **Variation Tip:** This recipe calls for rotini, but you can use any short cut pasta, such as penne. Long noodles like spaghetti and linguine tend to stick together in the Instant Pot.

Per Serving: Calories: 345; Fat: 6g; Protein: 24g; Carbohydrates: 46g; Fiber: 2.5g; Sugar: 3.5g; Sodium: 210mg

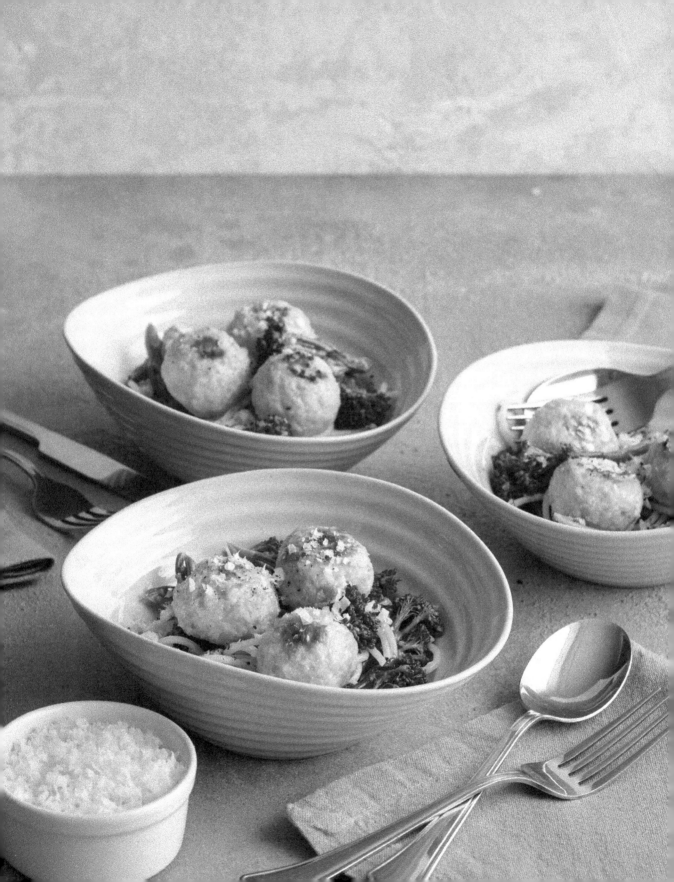

CHAPTER SIX

Poultry

Parmesan Turkey Meatballs

Serves 4

Prep time: 15 minutes / **Pressure cook:** 7 minutes on Sauté High; 5 minutes on High

Pressure release: Natural for 5 minutes, then Quick / **Total time:** 40 minutes

Parmesan cheese, garlic, and parsley flavor these easy turkey meatballs. They cook in a very plain tomato sauce, which lets the flavor of the meatballs shine through, but feel free to use a more complex homemade or store-bought sauce if you like. Try serving these over some whole wheat linguini and sautéed broccolini for a satisfyingly well-rounded meal.

---

1 pound ground turkey

1 small yellow onion, finely chopped

3 garlic cloves, minced

½ cup grated parmesan or similar cheese

2 tablespoons minced fresh parsley

½ teaspoon kosher salt

1 large egg

2 tablespoons whole milk

¼ cup plain bread crumbs

2 tablespoons extra-virgin olive oil

½ cup Chicken Stock (page 137) or store-bought low-sodium chicken stock

1 (14½-ounce) can diced tomatoes

1. In a large bowl, gently mix together the turkey, onion, garlic, cheese, parsley, and salt.

2. In a small bowl, whisk together the egg and milk. Stir in the bread crumbs.

3. Add the egg-crumb mixture to the turkey, and gently mix until just evenly combined.

4. Form meatballs using about 2 tablespoons of the mixture for each. You may find it easier to roll the balls if you moisten your hands with water.

5. Preheat the Instant Pot by selecting Sauté, and adjust to More for high heat.

6. Once hot, pour in the oil.

7. Add the meatballs in a single layer, and let cook undisturbed for 1 to 2 minutes, or until browned on the bottom. Turn to brown on the opposite side, then move to the sides of the pot (they may stack on top of each other).

8. Pour in the stock. Bring to a boil. Scrape up any browned bits from the bottom of the pot.

9. Add the tomatoes with their juices, and move the meatballs back into an even layer.

10. Lock the lid into place. Select Pressure Cook or Manual, and cook at High Pressure for 5 minutes.

11. After cooking, naturally release the pressure for 5 minutes, then quick release any remaining pressure.

12. Unlock and remove the lid. Using a slotted spoon, transfer the meatballs to a bowl.

13. Select Sauté, and adjust to More for high heat. Bring the sauce to a boil. Cook until very thick and chunky. Press Cancel to stop cooking.

14. Spoon the sauce over the meatballs, and serve.

Per Serving: Calories: 355; Fat: 20g; Protein: 30g; Carbohydrates: 14g; Fiber: 1.5g; Sugar: 4g; Sodium: 623mg

Stuffed Turkey Breast

Serves 6 to 8

Prep time: 20 minutes

Pressure cook: 6 minutes on Sauté Medium + 21 minutes on Sauté High; 25 minutes on High

Pressure release: Natural for 20 minutes / **Total time:** 1 hour 40 minutes

WORTH THE WAIT

Roasting a whole turkey can be tough to get right, but it can serve a big crowd. If you're feeding fewer than eight people, try a turkey breast filled with savory bread stuffing instead. Using your Instant Pot can free up the oven for side dishes. If you end up with extra stuffing, put it in a dish, and bake it to serve on the side. This will taste great any time of the year.

---

5 tablespoons unsalted butter, divided

1 large yellow onion, chopped

2 celery stalks, chopped

¾ cup chopped mushrooms

2 garlic cloves, minced

2 cups plain bread crumbs

2 tablespoons chopped fresh sage leaves

1 tablespoon chopped fresh parsley

¾ teaspoon kosher salt, plus more as needed

¼ teaspoon freshly ground black pepper, plus more as needed

3 cups Chicken Stock (page 137) or store-bought low-sodium chicken stock, divided

1 (2- to 3-pound) boneless, skinless turkey breast, butterflied to an even thickness

1. Preheat the Instant Pot by selecting Sauté.

2. Once hot, toss in 3 tablespoons of butter.

3. Once the butter has melted, add the onion and celery. Stir and cook for 3 minutes, or until the onion is translucent.

4. Add the mushrooms and garlic. Stir and cook for 3 minutes, or until the mushrooms are soft. Press Cancel to stop cooking. Transfer to a large bowl.

5. To the bowl, add the bread crumbs, sage, parsley, salt, and pepper. Mix.

6. Add the stock a bit at a time, and mix until you get a moist but crumbly texture, using ¾ to 1 cup of stock.

7. Lay the turkey breast, top-side down, on your work surface. If it isn't an even thickness, pound the thick parts until mostly even. Sprinkle with salt and pepper.

8. Spread the stuffing mixture on the breast, making it about as thick as the turkey breast itself, and leaving at least 1 inch on each side. Roll up tightly (but not so tightly that the stuffing squeezes out), and secure with kitchen twine. Season the outside of the breast with salt and pepper.

9. Preheat the Instant Pot by selecting Sauté, and adjust to More for high heat.

10. Once hot, toss in the remaining 2 tablespoons of butter.

11. Once melted, add the stuffed turkey, and brown on all sides, for about 3 minutes per side. Finish with it lying seam-side down in the pot.

12. Add the remaining 2 cups of stock.

13. Lock the lid into place. Select Pressure Cook or Manual, and cook at High Pressure for 25 minutes.

14. After cooking, naturally release the pressure for 15 to 20 minutes.

15. Unlock and remove the lid. Remove the turkey, and let rest, tented with aluminum foil.

16. Select Sauté, and adjust to More for high heat. To make the gravy, reduce the cooking liquid for 10 to 15 minutes, or until concentrated. Press Cancel to stop cooking.

17. Remove the kitchen twine from the turkey, and spoon the gravy over the top. Slice and serve.

❖ **Ingredient Tip:** When buying the turkey breast, have the butcher butterfly it for you to save time and effort. Just make sure it fits in your cooker first!

Per Serving: Calories: 401; Fat: 12g; Protein: 46g; Carbohydrates: 24g; Fiber: 3g; Sugar: 3.5g; Sodium: 530mg

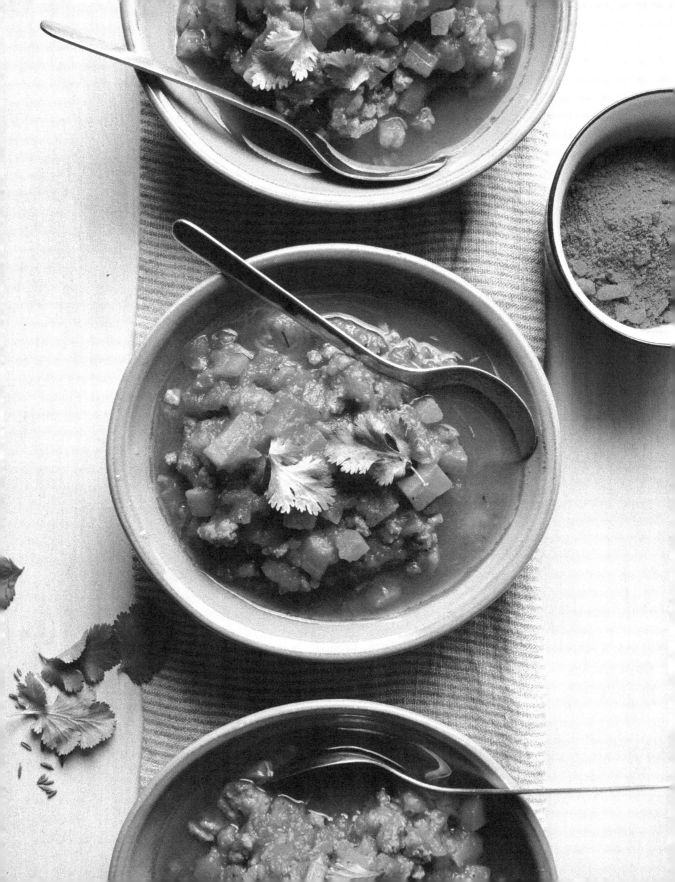

Sweet Potato and Ground Turkey Chili

Serves 8

Prep time: 10 minutes / **Pressure cook:** 2 minutes on Sauté; 10 minutes on High

Pressure release: Natural for 10 minutes, then Quick / **Total time:** 40 minutes

 ONE-POT MEAL

This bean-free chili has tons of flavor and heartiness from the ground turkey, vegetables, and sweet potato. The spices aren't too strong, so it's kid friendly as well. As delicious as this chili is, the leftovers taste even better than the first serving. It is perfect for potlucks, weeknight meals, or any time you want something easy, hearty, and delicious.

---

2 tablespoons extra-virgin olive oil

2 pounds ground turkey

3 medium sweet potatoes, peeled and cut into
　1-inch dice

1 medium yellow onion, diced

3 garlic cloves, minced

4 celery stalks, chopped

3 medium carrots, chopped

1 red bell pepper, cored and chopped

1 (14½-ounce) can diced tomatoes

3 cups Chicken Stock (page 137) or
　store-bought low-sodium chicken stock

½ teaspoon ground cumin

½ teaspoon chili powder

½ teaspoon kosher salt

Freshly ground black pepper

Chopped fresh cilantro, for garnish (optional)

1. Select Sauté, and pour the oil into the inner pot.

2. Once the oil is hot, add the turkey. Cook for 2 minutes, using a wooden spoon to break up the meat and keep it from sticking to the pot.

3. Press Cancel. Add the sweet potatoes, onion, garlic, celery, carrots, bell pepper, tomatoes with their juices, stock, cumin, and chili powder.

4. Lock the lid into place. Select Pressure Cook or Manual, and cook at High Pressure for 10 minutes.

5. After cooking, naturally release the pressure for 10 minutes, then quick release any remaining pressure.

6. Unlock and remove the lid. Stir in the salt and pepper.

7. Serve the chili immediately, garnished with cilantro (if using); refrigerate in an airtight container for up to 4 days; or freeze for up to 2 months.

❖ **Flavor Boost:** This chili goes really well with a few slices of fresh avocado per serving.

Per Serving: Calories: 287; Fat: 12g; Protein: 26g; Carbohydrates: 18g; Fiber: 3.5g; Sugar: 5.5g; Sodium: 327mg

TURKEY ENCHILADA SOUP

Serves 6

Prep time: 6 minutes / **Pressure cook:** 5 minutes on Sauté; 7 minutes on High
Pressure release: Quick / **Total time:** 25 minutes

ONE-POT MEAL   QUICK

The green chiles in this soup add a fiery punch, but if you don't want heat or are serving this to children, just use regular diced tomatoes for less spice. Top it with avocado slices and a squeeze of lime juice for a delicious soup that the whole family will enjoy.

1 tablespoon extra-virgin olive oil
1 medium yellow onion, diced
3 garlic cloves, minced
2 (10-ounce) cans diced tomatoes with
  green chiles
1 (15-ounce) can black beans, drained
  and rinsed
1 (10-ounce) can red enchilada sauce
2 cups shredded cooked turkey breast

4 cups Chicken Stock (page 137) or
  store-bought low-sodium chicken
  stock, divided
1 teaspoon ground cumin
¼ cup masa harina
8 ounces shredded sharp Cheddar cheese
Kosher salt
Freshly ground black pepper

1. Select Sauté, and pour the oil into the inner pot.

2. Once the oil is hot, add the onion and garlic. Sauté for 2 minutes.

3. Add the diced tomatoes with their juices, the beans, enchilada sauce, turkey, 3 cups of stock, and the cumin. Stir to combine.

4. Lock the lid into place. Select Pressure Cook or Manual, and cook at High Pressure for 7 minutes.

5. After cooking, quick release the pressure.

6. Unlock and remove the lid. In a bowl, whisk together the remaining 1 cup of stock and the masa harina.

7. Select Sauté, and bring the soup to a simmer. Then stir in the masa harina mixture for about 1 minute, or until the soup has thickened.

8. Slowly stir in the cheese until incorporated. Press Cancel to stop cooking.

9. Season the soup with salt and pepper.

♻ **Ingredient Tip:** Masa harina can usually be found in the Hispanic food section (or sometimes next to cornmeal) of most major grocery stores.

Per Serving: Calories: 415; Fat: 23g; Protein: 27g; Carbohydrates: 24g; Fiber: 6.5g; Sugar: 4.5g; Sodium: 1,452mg

TERIYAKI CHICKEN RICE BOWLS

Serves 4

Prep time: 10 minutes / **Pressure cook:** 8 minutes on High; 6 minutes on Sauté
Pressure release: Natural for 10 minutes, then Quick / **Total time:** 40 minutes

This recipe makes use of the helpful pot-in-pot method for the Instant Pot, in which one dish is cooked in the main insert and another is cooked on the steamer rack at the same time. Once you see how this works, you'll love how convenient and easy it is.

½ cup Chicken Stock (page 137) or
   store-bought low-sodium chicken stock
¼ cup reduced-sodium soy sauce
¼ cup brown sugar
1 tablespoon rice vinegar
2 garlic cloves, minced
1 teaspoon grated fresh ginger

1 pound boneless, skinless chicken thighs, cut
   into bite-size chunks
1½ cups long-grain rice, rinsed
1½ cups water
2 large bell peppers, cored and chopped
3 cups broccoli florets
1 tablespoon cornstarch
1 tablespoon cold water

1. Put the stock, soy sauce, sugar, vinegar, garlic, ginger, and chicken in the inner pot. Mix well.

2. Place a trivet inside the pot over the chicken mixture.

3. In a stainless steel cake pan or oven-safe bowl, combine the rice and water. Place over the trivet.

4. Lock the lid into place. Select Pressure Cook or Manual, and cook at High Pressure for 8 minutes.

5. After cooking, naturally release the pressure for 10 minutes, then quick release any remaining pressure.

6. Unlock and remove the lid. Carefully remove the steam rack with the rice.

7. Select Sauté, and add the bell peppers and broccoli. Simmer for about 5 minutes, or until the vegetables are crisp tender.

8. In a small bowl, whisk together the cornstarch and water. Add to the pot, and stir for 1 minute, or until the sauce has thickened. Press Cancel to stop cooking.

9. Serve the chicken and vegetables over rice.

❖ **Variation Tip:** Make this with chicken breast or extra-firm tofu using the same cooking time.

Per Serving: Calories: 491; Fat: 5g; Protein: 32g; Carbohydrates: 79g; Fiber: 3.5g; Sugar: 16g;
Sodium: 716mg

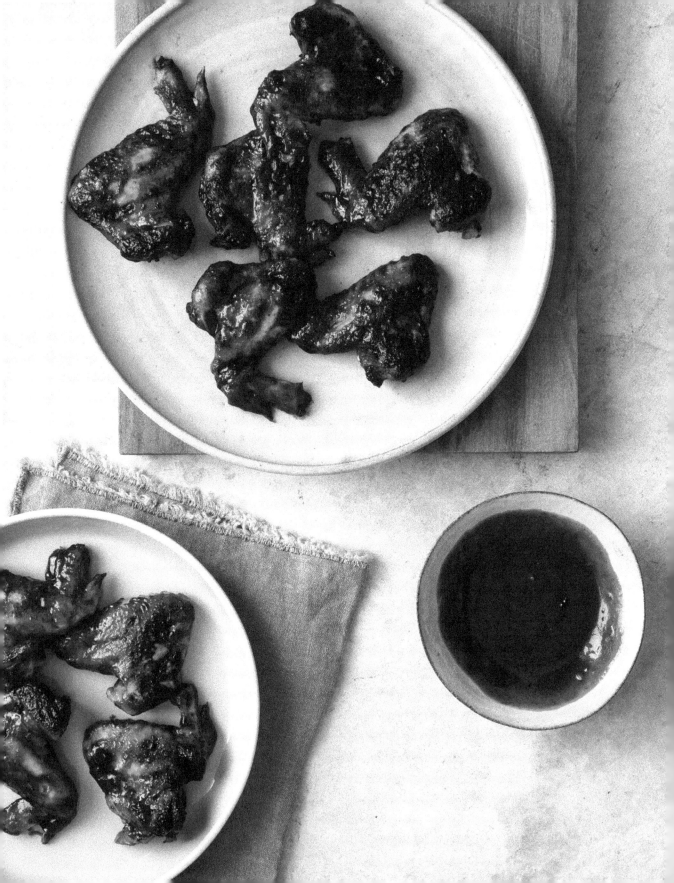

Sesame-Soy Chicken Wings

Serves 4

Prep time: 15 minutes / **Pressure cook:** 10 minutes on High; 3 minutes on Sauté High

Pressure release: Quick / **Total time:** 35 minutes

There's no denying that deep-frying chicken wings produces wonderful, crispy skin, but it's messy, time consuming, and not the healthiest. Instead, for velvety meat that practically falls off the bone, try braising your chicken wings in a savory soy-based broth. One taste, and you'll forget all about Buffalo wings!

12 whole chicken wings or 24 wing segments (drumettes, flats, or both)
1½ cups water, plus more as needed
½ cup reduced-sodium soy sauce
2 tablespoons toasted sesame oil
2 or 3 peeled ginger slices

3 garlic cloves, lightly smashed
2 tablespoons sugar
1 teaspoon Chinese five-spice powder
2 tablespoons minced fresh cilantro, basil leaves, or scallion greens

1. If you have whole wings, cut off the tips and discard. Cut each wing at the joint into a drumette and a flat segment.

2. Pour the water and soy sauce into the Instant Pot.

3. Add the oil, ginger, garlic, sugar, and five-spice powder. Stir to combine.

4. Add the wings, and stir to coat with the liquid. The wings should be mostly submerged. If necessary, add a little more water.

5. Lock the lid into place. Select Pressure Cook or Manual, and cook at High Pressure for 10 minutes.

6. After cooking, quick release the pressure.

7. Unlock and remove the lid. Using a spider or skimmer, remove the wings from the pot, and set aside on a plate.

8. Select Sauté, and adjust to More for high heat. Bring the liquid to a boil. Reduce by about half to make the sauce, about 3 minutes.

9. Return the wings to the sauce, and stir to coat. Press Cancel to stop cooking. Transfer the wings to a deep platter or bowl, and pour the sauce over.

10. Garnish with the cilantro, and serve.

Per Serving: Calories: 409; Fat: 27g; Protein: 31g; Carbohydrates: 9g; Fiber: 0.5g; Sugar: 6.5g; Sodium: 1,269mg

INDIAN-STYLE CHICKEN IN YOGURT SAUCE

Serves 4

Prep time: 20 minutes / **Pressure cook:** 8 minutes on High

Pressure release: Natural / **Total time:** 33 minutes

 ONE-POT MEAL

This chicken is based on an Indian tandoori-inspired dish in which chicken thighs marinate in spiced yogurt for several hours and are grilled or broiled. The cornstarch in the sauce keeps the yogurt from separating, so don't omit it. Add the cayenne pepper if you like a bit more heat in your chicken.

---

1 cup 2 percent plain Greek yogurt
1 teaspoon kosher salt
1 teaspoon ground ginger
1 teaspoon smoked or sweet paprika
1 teaspoon curry powder
1 teaspoon cornstarch
½ teaspoon ground turmeric
¼ teaspoon ground cayenne pepper (optional)
1¼ pounds boneless, skinless chicken thighs (4 to 6 thighs), trimmed of excess fat
Cooked brown or white rice, for serving

1. In the Instant Pot, stir together the yogurt, salt, ginger, paprika, curry powder, cornstarch, turmeric, and cayenne pepper (if using). Let the sauce sit for 5 minutes so the cornstarch hydrates fully.

2. Add the chicken, and stir to coat. Distribute in a single layer as much as possible.

3. Lock the lid into place. Select Pressure Cook or Manual, and cook at High Pressure for 8 minutes.

4. After cooking, naturally release the pressure.

5. Unlock and remove the lid. Serve the chicken and sauce over rice.

Per Serving (without rice): Calories: 212; Fat: 6.5g; Protein: 35g; Carbohydrates: 3g; Fiber: 0g; Sugar: 2g; Sodium: 424mg

Duck with Mushrooms and Onions

Serves 4

Prep time: 10 minutes

Pressure cook: 5 minutes on Sauté High + 7 minutes on Sauté Medium; 20 minutes on High

Pressure release: Quick / **Total time:** 42 minutes

 ONE-POT MEAL

Duck meat is darker, richer, and juicier than chicken. First, duck legs are seared to create a crispy skin and release some of the excess fat. Then they are cooked until tender with mushrooms, onions, and wine. Make this dish for a special occasion—it's sure to impress.

2 tablespoons vegetable oil	8 ounces sliced mushrooms
4 duck legs	4 garlic cloves, minced
Kosher salt	½ cup dry red wine
Freshly ground pepper	1 cup Chicken Stock (page 137) or store-bought
8 ounces small cipolline or pearl onions	low-sodium chicken stock

1. Preheat the Instant Pot by selecting Sauté, and adjust to More for high heat. Pour in the oil.

2. Dry the duck well. Season with salt and pepper. Place, skin-side down, in the pot, and cook for about 5 minutes, or until nicely browned. Remove to a plate.

3. Reduce the heat to medium. Carefully discard all but 2 tablespoons of the fat and oil in the pot.

4. Add the onions, and sauté for about 3 minutes, or until lightly browned.

5. Add the mushrooms and garlic. Cook, stirring, for 3 minutes.

6. Add the wine, and scrape up any brown bits off the bottom of the pot, cooking for 1 minute.

7. Add the stock and duck.

8. Lock the lid into place. Select Pressure Cook or Manual, and cook at High Pressure for 20 minutes.

9. After cooking, quick release the pressure.

10. Unlock and remove the lid. Serve the duck with the onions and mushrooms, and spoon over some of the cooking liquid.

Per Serving: Calories: 303; Fat: 14g; Protein: 29g; Carbohydrates: 9g; Fiber: 1.5g; Sugar: 3.5g; Sodium: 212mg

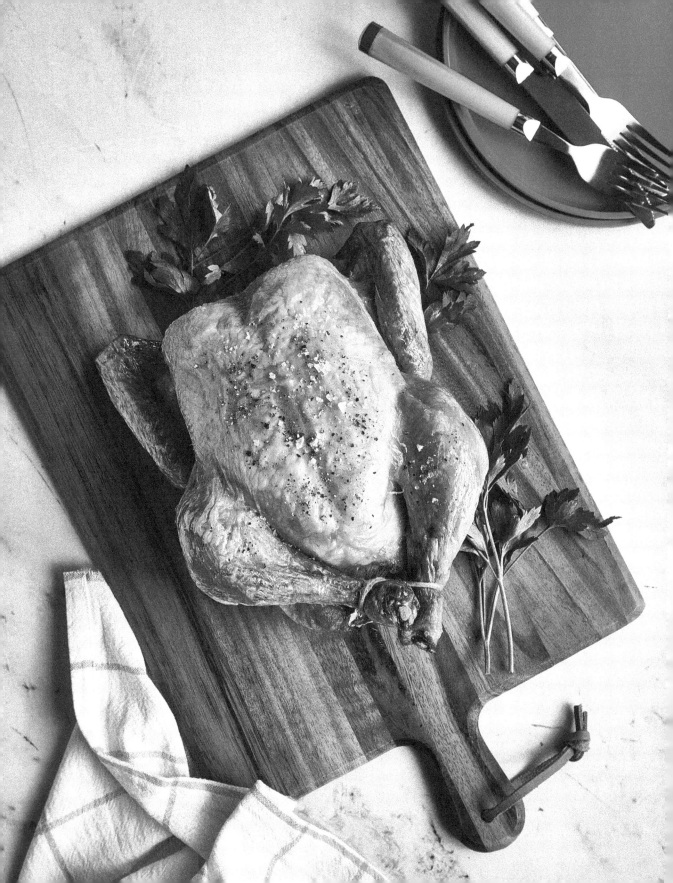

WHOLE CHICKEN

Serves 6

Prep time: 5 minutes / **Pressure cook:** 10 minutes on Sauté High; 30 minutes on High
Pressure release: Natural for 15 minutes, then Quick / **Total time:** 1 hour 10 minutes

 5 OR FEWER INGREDIENTS **WORTH THE WAIT**

There's something cozy about a juicy, tender whole chicken. Searing helps lock in the flavor and gives it a golden brown hue, making it look even more appetizing. Feel free to swap out the herbs for whatever you like and have on hand. Serve with Garlicky Lemon Broccoli (page 41) or Lemon-Ginger Asparagus (page 43).

---

1 (3- to 4-pound) whole chicken,
  giblets removed
2 teaspoons kosher salt
1 teaspoon freshly ground black pepper

1 tablespoon extra-virgin olive oil
½ cup water
6 garlic cloves, peeled
1 bunch fresh rosemary, thyme, parsley, or sage

1. Season the chicken with the salt and pepper.

2. Preheat the Instant Pot by selecting Sauté, and adjust to More for high heat.

3. Once hot, pour in the oil.

4. Add the chicken, breast-side down, and cook for 5 minutes undisturbed. Using tongs or 2 large spoons, carefully turn the chicken over, and cook for 5 minutes, or until browned.

5. Add the water, carefully drop in the garlic, and lay the herbs around and across the top of the chicken.

6. Lock the lid into place. Select Pressure Cook or Manual, and cook at High Pressure for 30 minutes.

7. After cooking, naturally release the pressure for 15 minutes, then quick release any remaining pressure. Unlock and remove the lid. Transfer the chicken to a large cutting board. Let rest for another 10 minutes, then cut and serve.

♻ **Ingredient Tip:** Leftover chicken has endless possibilities! Add it to soups, stew, salads, sandwiches, grain bowls, and more. It will keep in the refrigerator for up to 4 days.

Per Serving: Calories: 314; Fat: 18g; Protein: 34g; Carbohydrates: 0g; Fiber: 0g; Sugar: 0g; Sodium: 103mg

Chicken Cacciatore

Serves 5

Prep time: 5 minutes / **Pressure cook:** 8 minutes on Sauté; 12 minutes on High

Pressure release: Natural / **Total time:** 45 minutes

 ONE-POT MEAL

Juicy chicken thighs are cooked in a tasty tomato sauce flavored with vegetables, herbs, and olives. It's simple, rustic, and wholesome. Like all stews, this dish tastes even better the next day!

2 pounds boneless, skinless chicken thighs	1 medium yellow onion, diced	½ cup green olives, halved	2 tablespoons tomato paste
Kosher salt	3 garlic cloves, minced	1 (15-ounce) can crushed tomatoes	1 bay leaf
Freshly ground black pepper	1 large green bell pepper, cored and diced	½ cup Chicken Stock (page 137) or store-bought low-sodium chicken stock	1 rosemary sprig
1 tablespoon extra-virgin olive oil	2 cups sliced mushrooms		

1. Season the chicken with salt and pepper.

2. Select Sauté, and pour the oil into the inner pot.

3. Once the oil is hot, add the chicken, and brown for 3 minutes per side. Remove to a plate.

4. Add the onion and garlic to the pot, and sauté for 2 minutes.

5. Add the chicken, bell pepper, mushrooms, olives, tomatoes, stock, tomato paste, bay leaf, and rosemary.

6. Lock the lid into place. Select Pressure Cook or Manual, and cook at High Pressure for 12 minutes.

7. After cooking, naturally release the pressure.

8. Unlock and remove the lid. Remove and discard the bay leaf and rosemary. Season with salt and pepper.

♻ **Serving Tip:** While not gluten-free, serving this with crusty garlic bread is pretty tasty.

Per Serving: Calories: 320; Fat: 11g; Protein: 41g; Carbohydrates: 13g; Fiber: 4g; Sugar: 6g; Sodium: 644mg

CAPRESE CHICKEN

Serves 4

Prep time: 5 minutes / **Pressure cook:** 8 minutes on Sauté; 3 minutes on High

Pressure release: Quick / **Total time:** 25 minutes

 ONE-POT MEAL QUICK

This chicken dish is bursting with flavors reminiscent of a caprese salad, with ripe tomatoes, fresh basil, mozzarella cheese, and balsamic glaze. It's a comforting reminder of warm summer days and perfect for any night of the week, all year.

1½ pounds boneless, skinless chicken breasts
Kosher salt
Freshly ground black pepper
1 tablespoon extra-virgin olive oil
2 shallots, sliced
2 garlic cloves, minced
3½ cups cherry or grape tomatoes, halved

¼ cup Chicken Stock (page 137) or store-bought low-sodium chicken stock
2 tablespoons tomato paste
½ teaspoon red pepper flakes (optional)
6 ounces fresh mozzarella cheese, sliced
2 tablespoons balsamic glaze
¼ cup chopped fresh basil leaves

1. Season the chicken with salt and pepper.

2. Select Sauté, and pour the oil into the inner pot.

3. Once the oil is hot, add the chicken, and brown for 3 minutes per side. Remove to a plate.

4. Add the shallots and garlic to the pot, and sauté for 2 minutes.

5. Add the chicken, tomatoes, stock, tomato paste, and red pepper flakes (if using).

6. Lock the lid into place. Select Pressure Cook or Manual, and cook at High Pressure for 3 minutes.

7. After cooking, quick release the pressure.

8. Unlock and remove the lid. Season the chicken with salt and pepper. Top with the mozzarella slices, and cover with the lid (but don't lock it in place) to let the cheese melt.

9. Drizzle the balsamic glaze over the chicken, and garnish with the basil before serving.

♻ **Ingredient Tip:** Instead of fresh mozzarella slices, you can use the same amount of shredded mozzarella cheese.

Per Serving: Calories: 402; Fat: 15g; Protein: 48g; Carbohydrates: 15g; Fiber: 2.5g; Sugar: 7g; Sodium: 300mg

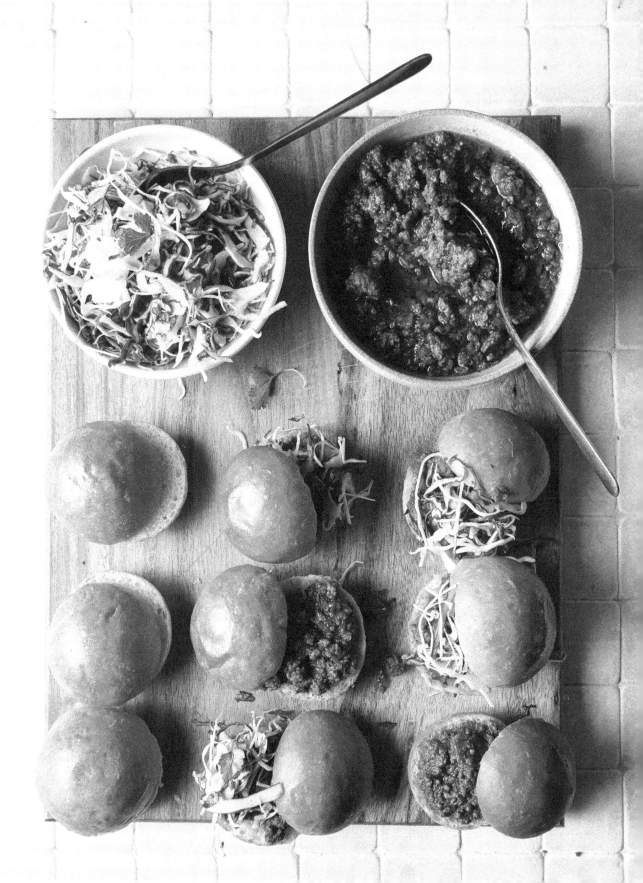

CHAPTER SEVEN

Beef and Pork

Sloppy Joes

Serves 8

Prep time: 5 minutes / **Pressure cook:** 3 minutes on Sauté; 10 minutes on High
Pressure release: Natural for 10 minutes, then Quick / **Total time:** 35 minutes

 ONE-POT MEAL

These Sloppy Joes are perfect for those evenings when you don't have anything planned but need dinner on the table fast. You just add the meat and spices and let the Instant Pot do all the work. Try serving these on hamburger buns or, for a healthier option, on top of Garlic-Herb Mashed Potatoes (page 47) or Cilantro-Lime Rice (page 44).

---

1 tablespoon extra-virgin olive oil
2 pounds 90 percent lean ground beef
1 (16-ounce) can tomato puree
½ cup ketchup
2 tablespoons reduced-sodium soy sauce
1 tablespoon brown sugar

1 teaspoon onion powder
1 teaspoon chili powder
½ teaspoon garlic powder
Coleslaw, for garnish (optional)
Fresh chopped parsley, for garnish (optional)

1. Select Sauté, and pour the oil into the inner pot.

2. Once the oil is hot, add the beef, and cook, using a spatula to break up the meat, for 3 minutes.

3. Add the tomato puree, ketchup, soy sauce, sugar, onion powder, chili powder, and garlic powder. Stir to combine.

4. Lock the lid into place. Select Pressure Cook or Manual, and cook at High Pressure for 10 minutes.

5. After cooking, naturally release the pressure for 10 minutes, then quick release any remaining pressure.

6. Unlock and remove the lid. Serve the Sloppy Joes immediately, garnished with coleslaw (if using) and parsley (if using); refrigerate in an airtight container for up to 4 days; or freeze for up to 2 months.

❖ **Substitution Tip:** To make this gluten-free, use tamari in place of the soy sauce.

Per Serving: Calories: 265; Fat: 13g; Protein: 24g; Carbohydrates: 12g; Fiber: 1g; Sugar: 8.5g; Sodium: 494mg

FIVE-SPICE BONELESS BEEF RIBS

Serves 6

Prep time: 15 minutes / **Pressure cook:** 10 minutes on Sauté High; 35 minutes on High

Pressure release: Natural for 15 minutes / **Total time:** 1 hour 30 minutes

 WORTH THE WAIT

Serve these tender and flavorful ribs over steamed rice.

---

6 boneless beef short ribs, trimmed

2 teaspoons Chinese five-spice powder

Kosher salt

2 tablespoons canola oil

4 garlic cloves, minced

1 (1-inch) piece fresh ginger, finely chopped

2 tablespoons rice vinegar

½ cup low-sodium beef stock

¼ cup reduced-sodium soy sauce

¼ cup brown sugar

1. Preheat the oven to broil.

2. Coat the ribs with the five-spice powder. Season with salt. Transfer to a baking sheet.

3. Transfer the baking sheet to the oven, and broil the ribs for 3 minutes per side. Remove from the oven.

4. Preheat the Instant Pot by selecting Sauté High, and pour in the oil.

5. Once the oil is hot, add the garlic and ginger. Sauté for 2 minutes, or until starting to brown.

6. Add the vinegar, and cook for 1 minute.

7. Press Cancel, and add the stock, soy sauce, and sugar. Stir until the sugar dissolves.

8. Add the ribs.

9. Lock the lid into place. Select Pressure Cook or Manual, and cook at High Pressure for 35 minutes.

10. After cooking, naturally release the pressure for 15 minutes.

11. Unlock and remove the lid. Remove the ribs, and put back on the baking sheet.

12. Brush with the cooking liquid. Transfer the baking sheet to the oven, and broil again for 3 minutes per side to form a crust. Remove from the oven.

13. Meanwhile, select Sauté, and adjust to More for high heat. Reduce the cooking liquid by up to half to make the sauce.

14. After broiling, brush the ribs on all sides with the sauce. Serve with extra sauce.

Per Serving: Calories: 378; Fat: 22g; Protein: 32g; Carbohydrates: 10g; Fiber: 0g; Sugar: 9g; Sodium: 497mg

Hearty Beef Chili

Serves 8

Prep time: 10 minutes / **Pressure cook:** 3 minutes on Sauté; 10 minutes on High

Pressure release: Natural for 10 minutes, then Quick / **Total time:** 40 minutes

 ONE-POT MEAL

Stovetop chili, begone. Just add everything to the Instant Pot, walk away, and let it do all of the work. It's a favorite for potlucks, game days, or any time you want to serve a crowd. This version is not too spicy, with a rich tomato flavor and a hint of sweetness from the Worcestershire sauce.

2 tablespoons extra-virgin olive oil

2 pounds 90 percent lean ground beef

1 medium yellow onion, diced

3 garlic cloves, minced

1 teaspoon chili powder

½ teaspoon ground cumin

4 cups low-sodium beef stock

1 (28-ounce) can crushed tomatoes

1 (15-ounce) can kidney beans, drained and rinsed

1 teaspoon Worcestershire sauce

1. Select Sauté, and pour the oil into the inner pot.

2. Once the oil is hot, add the beef, onion, garlic, chili powder, and cumin. Cook for 3 minutes, or until the beef starts to brown.

3. Pour in the stock. Using a wooden spoon, scrape up any browned bits stuck to the bottom of the pot.

4. Add the tomatoes and beans, but don't stir.

5. Lock the lid into place. Select Pressure Cook or Manual, and cook at High Pressure for 10 minutes.

6. After cooking, naturally release the pressure for 10 minutes, then quick release any remaining pressure.

7. Unlock and remove the lid. Stir in the Worcestershire sauce.

8. Serve the chili immediately, refrigerate in an airtight container for up to 4 days, or freeze for up to 2 months.

✿ **Variation Tip:** Instead of kidney beans, you can use canned white beans, black beans, or navy beans.

Per Serving: Calories: 330; Fat: 14g; Protein: 29g; Carbohydrates: 19g; Fiber: 4.5g; Sugar: 6.5g; Sodium: 467mg

BEEF STEW WITH ROOT VEGETABLES

Serves 6

Prep time: 5 minutes / **Pressure cook:** 13 minutes on Sauté; 30 minutes on High

Pressure release: Natural for 10 minutes, then Quick / **Total time:** 1 hour 5 minutes

 ONE-POT MEAL WORTH THE WAIT

This hearty beef stew is perfect for family dinner or when company is over, since you can just set it and forget it without having to worry about watching the stove.

1½ pounds beef chuck roast, cut into 1-inch dice
1 teaspoon kosher salt, plus more as needed
½ teaspoon freshly ground black pepper, plus more as needed
2 tablespoons extra-virgin olive oil
1 medium yellow onion, diced
2 garlic cloves, minced
3 medium carrots, chopped
2 parsnips, peeled and chopped

2 Yukon Gold or red potatoes, cut into 1-inch pieces
4 thyme sprigs
1 rosemary sprig
2 cups low-sodium beef stock
2 tablespoons tomato paste
1 tablespoon water
2 teaspoons cornstarch
¼ cup chopped fresh parsley

1. Season the beef with the salt and pepper.

2. Select Sauté, and pour the oil into the inner pot.

3. Once the oil is hot, add the beef, and brown for 5 minutes per side. Transfer to a plate.

4. Add the onion and garlic to the pot, and sauté for 2 minutes.

5. Add the carrots, parsnips, potatoes, thyme, rosemary, stock, and tomato paste.

6. Lock the lid into place. Select Pressure Cook or Manual, and cook at High Pressure for 30 minutes.

7. After cooking, naturally release the pressure for 10 minutes, then quick release any remaining pressure.

8. Unlock and remove the lid. Remove and discard the thyme and rosemary.

9. In a small bowl, whisk together the water and cornstarch.

10. Select Sauté. Once the liquid is simmering, stir in the cornstarch mixture, and simmer for about 1 minute, or until the sauce has thickened. Press Cancel to stop cooking. Season with salt and pepper.

11. Garnish with the parsley before serving.

Per Serving: Calories: 277; Fat: 10g; Protein: 27g; Carbohydrates: 21g; Fiber: 3g; Sugar: 4.5g; Sodium: 356mg

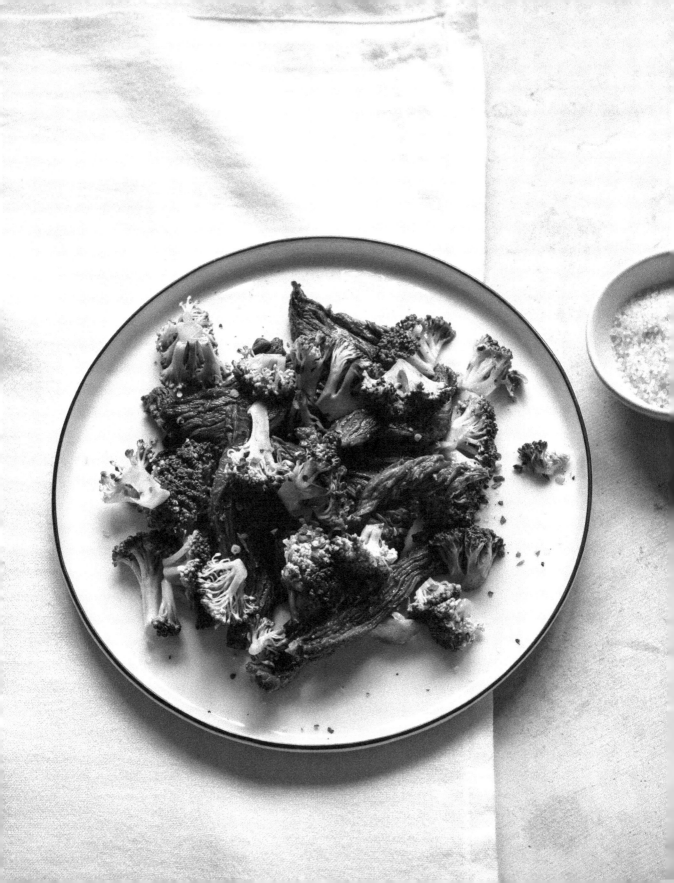

Ginger Beef and Broccoli

Serves 4

Prep time: 9 minutes / **Pressure cook:** 8 minutes on Sauté; 10 minutes on High

Pressure release: Quick / **Total time:** 35 minutes

 ONE-POT MEAL

Skip the takeout, and make this delicious Asian-inspired dish that is guaranteed to become one of your go-to weeknight dinners. Not a fan of broccoli? You can use pretty much any vegetables you want, such as cauliflower, baby corn, snap peas, or carrots.

2 tablespoons vegetable oil	½ cup reduced-sodium soy sauce
1½ pounds boneless beef chuck, trimmed and sliced	⅓ cup packed brown sugar
4 garlic cloves, minced	1 teaspoon sesame oil
1 teaspoon grated fresh ginger	⅛ teaspoon red pepper flakes
¾ cup water, divided	4 cups broccoli florets
	2 tablespoons cornstarch

1. Select Sauté, and pour the vegetable oil into the inner pot.

2. Once the oil is hot, add the beef, and brown for 3 minutes.

3. Add the garlic and ginger. Cook for 1 minute.

4. Add ½ cup of water, the soy sauce, sugar, sesame oil, and red pepper flakes. Stir to combine.

5. Lock the lid into place. Select Pressure Cook or Manual, and cook at High Pressure for 10 minutes.

6. After cooking, quick release the pressure.

7. Unlock and remove the lid. Select Sauté. Once the liquid is simmering, stir in the broccoli, and cook for 3 minutes, or until crisp tender.

8. In a bowl, whisk together the cornstarch and remaining ¼ cup of water.

9. Add the cornstarch mixture to the pot, and simmer for about 1 minute, or until the sauce has thickened. Press Cancel to stop cooking.

❖ **Ingredient Tip:** Frozen broccoli florets can be substituted for fresh broccoli. Defrost and drain well before adding them to the pot.

Per Serving: Calories: 420; Fat: 17g; Protein: 42g; Carbohydrates: 28g; Fiber: 2g; Sugar: 19g; Sodium: 1,311mg

→

BEEF BURGUNDY

Serves 8

Prep time: 10 minutes / **Pressure cook:** 3 minutes on Sauté; 30 minutes on High

Pressure release: Natural for 10 minutes, then Quick / **Total time:** 1 hour

 WORTH THE WAIT

It's impossible not to love this dish once you see how easy it is to throw together. The red wine creates a rich, elegant sauce that coats the beef and infuses every bite with robust flavor. This dish goes nicely with steamed broccoli or cauliflower and a baked potato on the side.

---

2 pounds beef chuck roast, cut into 1-inch dice
¼ cup all-purpose flour
2 tablespoons extra-virgin olive oil
2 garlic cloves, minced
1 medium yellow onion, diced
1 teaspoon dried thyme

1 teaspoon kosher salt
½ teaspoon freshly ground black pepper
1 cup dry red wine
1 tablespoon tomato paste
4 medium carrots, sliced

1. Put the beef and flour in a zip-top bag. Seal the bag, and shake to coat the beef with the flour.

2. Select Sauté, and pour the oil into the inner pot.

3. Once the oil is hot, add the flour-coated beef, garlic, onion, thyme, salt, and pepper. Sauté, stirring occasionally, for 3 minutes.

4. Pour in the wine. Using a wooden spoon, scrape up any browned bits stuck to the bottom of the pot.

5. Add the tomato paste and carrots. Stir to combine.

6. Lock the lid into place. Select Pressure Cook or Manual, and cook at High Pressure for 30 minutes.

7. After cooking, naturally release the pressure for 10 minutes, then quick release any remaining pressure.

8. Unlock and remove the lid. Serve the beef and sauce immediately, refrigerate in an airtight container for up to 4 days, or freeze for up to 2 months.

♻ **Ingredient Tip:** To make this gluten-free, use your favorite gluten-free flour blend instead of all-purpose flour. Also, make sure the tomato paste is gluten-free. Some brands are processed with gluten products.

Per Serving: Calories: 234; Fat: 9g; Protein: 25g; Carbohydrates: 8g; Fiber: 1g; Sugar: 2g; Sodium: 253mg

HOISIN BEEF LETTUCE WRAPS

Serves 4

Prep time: 5 minutes / **Pressure cook:** 5 minutes on Sauté; 2 minutes on High

Pressure release: Quick / **Total time:** 20 minutes

 ONE-POT MEAL QUICK

These lettuce wraps are the perfect blend of sweet and savory and come together quickly with the help of a few basic pantry staples. I like to use butter lettuce because it has a nice crispness, is easy to roll, and is firm enough to hold all the filling without tearing. If you like a bit of heat, try adding a teaspoon of chili-garlic sauce or sriracha to the dish.

2 teaspoons sesame oil

1 pound 90 percent lean ground beef

2 garlic cloves, minced

1 teaspoon grated fresh ginger

1 (8-ounce) can water chestnuts, drained and finely chopped

1 medium carrot, diced

¼ cup hoisin sauce

¼ cup water

1 tablespoon reduced-sodium soy sauce

1 tablespoon rice vinegar

1 head butter lettuce, leaves separated, washed, and dried

2 tablespoons chopped scallions, green parts only

1. Select Sauté, and pour the oil into the inner pot.

2. Once the oil is hot, add the beef, and brown for 4 minutes.

3. Add the garlic and ginger. Cook for 1 minute.

4. Add the water chestnuts, carrot, hoisin sauce, water, soy sauce, and vinegar. Stir to combine.

5. Lock the lid into place. Select Pressure Cook or Manual, and cook at High Pressure for 2 minutes.

6. After cooking, quick release the pressure.

7. Unlock and remove the lid. Arrange the lettuce leaves on a serving platter, and pile the meat mixture in the center.

8. Garnish with the scallions before serving.

Flavor Boost: For extra crunch and nutty flavor, garnish the lettuce wraps with crushed roasted peanuts or cashews.

Per Serving: Calories: 283; Fat: 14g; Protein: 25g; Carbohydrates: 13g; Fiber: 2.5g; Sugar: 6g; Sodium: 493mg

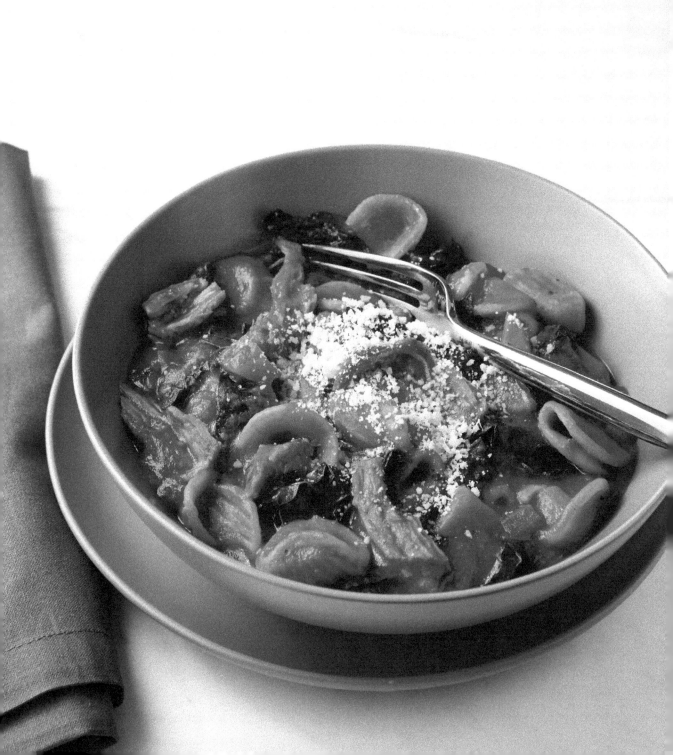

Pork Ragù

Serves 4

Prep time: 15 minutes / **Pressure cook:** 9 minutes on Sauté; 45 minutes on High
Pressure release: Natural for 15 minutes, then Quick / **Total time:** 1 hour 35 minutes

 ONE-POT MEAL   WORTH THE WAIT

A pork shoulder can also be used for a richer ragù; just be sure to adjust the amounts of the other ingredients accordingly based on the size of the cut. Serve this dish over pasta, vegetable noodles, or whole grains, such as brown rice.

---

1 pound pork tenderloin
1 teaspoon kosher salt
½ teaspoon freshly ground black pepper
2 tablespoons extra-virgin olive oil, divided
1 large white onion, diced
5 garlic cloves, minced

½ cup dry white wine
1 (28-ounce) can low-sodium whole tomatoes
½ cup low-sodium vegetable stock
1 tablespoon Italian seasoning
½ teaspoon fennel seeds
¼ teaspoon red pepper flakes

1. Season the pork with the salt and pepper.

2. Preheat the Instant Pot by selecting Sauté.

3. Once hot, pour in 1 tablespoon of oil.

4. Add the pork, and cook for about 3 minutes on each side, or until browned. Remove the pork to a plate.

5. Heat the remaining 1 tablespoon of oil. Add the onion, and sauté for 2 minutes, or until softened. Add the garlic, and sauté for 30 seconds, or until fragrant.

6. Add the wine, and deglaze: mix well, and scrape up any brown bits on the bottom of the pot.

7. Add the tomatoes with their juices, the stock, Italian seasoning, fennel seeds, and red pepper flakes. Mix well.

8. Return the pork to the pot. Lock the lid into place. Select Pressure Cook or Manual, and cook at High Pressure for 45 minutes.

9. After cooking, naturally release the pressure for 15 minutes, then quick release any remaining pressure.

10. Unlock and remove the lid. Using two forks, shred the pork. Serve.

❖ **Ingredient Tip:** Put leftovers in an airtight container, and refrigerate for up to 5 days, or freeze for up to 3 months.

Per Serving: Calories: 305; Carbohydrates: 19g; Fat: 11g; Fiber: 4g; Protein: 26g; Sugar: 12g; Sodium: 410mg

Pork Tenderloin with Rice Pilaf

Serves 4

Prep time: 15 minutes, plus 2 hours to brine (optional)

Pressure cook: 10 minutes on Sauté; 5 minutes on High

Pressure release: Quick / **Total time:** 2 hours 45 minutes

 ONE-POT MEAL   WORTH THE WAIT

The USDA has finally confirmed what countless chefs have suspected for years: pork is perfectly safe cooked to 145°F. Pork tenderloin, especially, is certainly more delicious with a hint of pink in the center. It stays juicy and tender, and brining increases that effect. Don't worry that the pork will be too salty; it absorbs just enough salt to season the meat to the center.

FOR THE BRINE (OPTIONAL)

½ cup kosher salt

¼ cup sugar

2 cups very hot tap water

2 cups ice water

FOR THE PORK AND RICE

1 (1-pound) pork tenderloin, trimmed of silverskin and halved

½ teaspoon kosher salt, plus more as needed

2 tablespoons extra-virgin olive oil

½ cup chopped onion

¼ cup chopped red bell pepper

¼ cup chopped green bell pepper

1 large garlic clove, minced

¾ cup long-grain white rice

1½ cups plus 2 tablespoons low-sodium vegetable stock or chicken stock

⅔ cup frozen green peas, thawed

TO MAKE THE BRINE (IF USING)

1. In a large stainless steel or glass bowl, dissolve the salt and sugar in the hot water, then stir in the ice water.

TO MAKE THE PORK AND RICE

2. Submerge the pork in the brine, and refrigerate for 2 to 3 hours. Drain, and pat dry. If you choose not to brine the pork, sprinkle liberally with kosher salt.

3. Select Sauté, and pour the oil into the inner pot.

4. Once the oil is hot, add the pork, and brown on all sides for about 4 minutes total. Transfer to a plate or rack.

5. Add the onion, red bell pepper, green bell pepper, and garlic to the pot. Cook, stirring occasionally, for about 2 minutes, or until the onion pieces separate and the vegetables soften.

6. Add the rice, and stir briefly just to coat with the oil.

7. Add the stock and ½ teaspoon of salt. Bring to a simmer. Stir to make sure the rice isn't clumping, and cook for 1 minute. Return the pork to the pot.

8. Lock the lid into place. Select Pressure Cook or Manual, and cook at High Pressure for 5 minutes.

9. After cooking, quick release the pressure.

10. Unlock and remove the lid. Quickly remove the pork to a plate or rack. Cover loosely with aluminum foil.

11. Stir the peas into the rice. Replace but *do not lock* the lid. Let the rice steam for 8 minutes.

12. Slice the pork against the grain. When the rice is steamed, fluff lightly with a fork, and serve with the pork.

❖ **Flavor Boost:** For a southwestern version, sprinkle the tenderloin with chili powder, and add 1 chopped jalapeño pepper and 1 chopped poblano pepper to the vegetable mixture in step 5.

Per Serving: Calories: 348; Fat: 9.5g; Protein: 28g; Carbohydrates: 35g; Fiber: 2.5g; Sugar: 3g; Sodium: 136mg

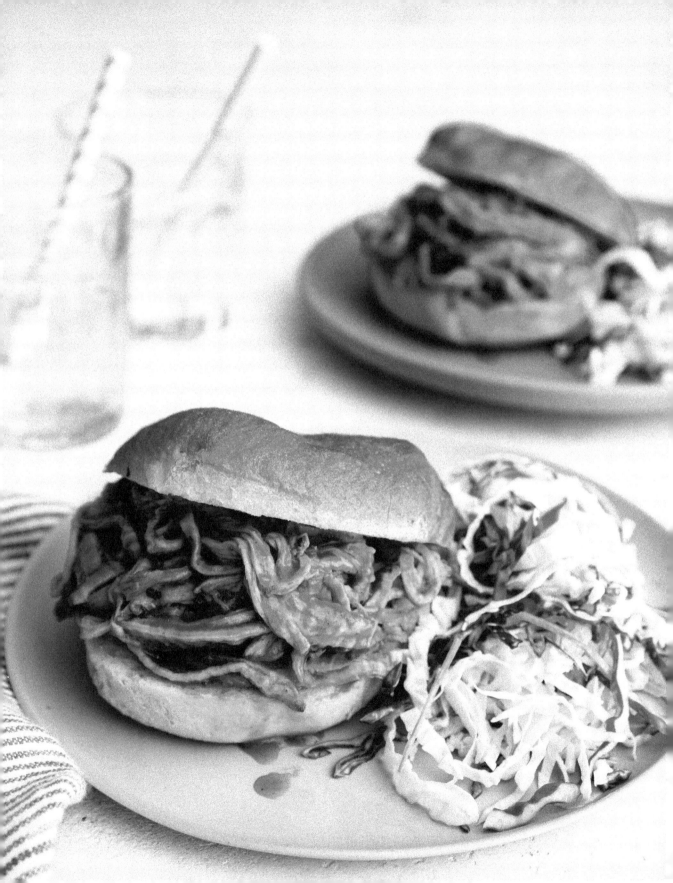

Pulled Pork with Mustardy Barbecue Sauce

Serves 4

Prep time: 5 minutes / **Pressure cook:** 25 minutes on High; 5 minutes on Sauté
Pressure release: Natural / **Total time:** 45 minutes

 ONE-POT MEAL

True pulled pork is a masterpiece, but it takes hours and hours over low heat and smoke. It's the perfect order at a barbecue restaurant but can be a lot of work to make at home. This cheater's version can be made—and enjoyed—on a weeknight, so that counts for a lot. Serve on whole wheat buns with a side of coleslaw and you have a full meal ready to eat.

6 tablespoons ketchup
2 tablespoons yellow mustard
2 tablespoons Dijon mustard
2 tablespoons honey
1 tablespoon apple cider vinegar
1 teaspoon Worcestershire sauce

1 teaspoon ground cayenne pepper
½ teaspoon kosher salt
1½ pounds boneless pork shoulder, trimmed of as much visible fat as possible, cut into 2-inch chunks
Buns or lettuce leaves, for serving (optional)

1. In the inner pot, stir together the ketchup, yellow mustard, Dijon mustard, honey, vinegar, Worcestershire sauce, cayenne, and salt until thoroughly mixed.

2. Add the pork, and toss to coat.

3. Lock the lid into place. Select Pressure Cook or Manual, and cook at High Pressure for 25 minutes.

4. After cooking, naturally release the pressure.

5. Unlock and remove the lid. Pour the pork and sauce through a coarse sieve; set the pork aside to cool. Return the sauce to the cooker, and let sit for 1 to 2 minutes so any fat rises to the surface. Skim or blot off as much fat as possible, and discard.

6. Press Sauté, and allow the Instant Pot to heat up. Simmer the sauce for about 5 minutes, or until the consistency of a thick tomato sauce.

7. While the sauce thickens, shred the pork, discarding any fat or gristle.

8. Add the shredded pork to the sauce, and heat through. Press Cancel to stop cooking. Serve on buns (if using), or use as a filling for lettuce wraps.

Per Serving: Calories: 399; Fat: 21g; Protein: 32g; Carbohydrates: 16g; Fiber: 0g; Sugar: 14g; Sodium: 799mg

Balsamic-Glazed Pork Tenderloin

Serves 6

Prep time: 5 minutes / **Pressure cook:** 10 minutes on Sauté; 15 minutes on High

Pressure release: Natural for 10 minutes, then Quick / **Total time:** 50 minutes

 WORTH THE WAIT

When my husband saw me putting the pork tenderloin in the Instant Pot, he had serious doubts. Wouldn't it turn out tough and dry? Not at all. In fact, it was tender, juicy, and absolutely delicious with the sweet, tangy balsamic glaze. It has become a dish we make on a regular basis, without a doubt!

---

2 to 2½ pounds pork tenderloin
Kosher salt
Freshly ground black pepper
2 tablespoons extra-virgin olive oil
½ cup packed brown sugar
½ cup water, divided

¼ cup balsamic vinegar
3 tablespoons reduced-sodium soy sauce
3 garlic cloves, minced
2 teaspoons Italian seasoning
2 tablespoons cornstarch

1. Season the pork with salt and pepper.

2. Select Sauté, and pour the oil into the inner pot.

3. Once the oil is hot, add the pork, and cook, turning over every 1 to 2 minutes, until browned on all sides.

4. Add the sugar, ¼ cup of water, the vinegar, soy sauce, garlic, and Italian seasoning. Stir to combine.

5. Lock the lid into place. Select Pressure Cook or Manual, and cook at High Pressure for 15 minutes.

6. After cooking, naturally release the pressure for 10 minutes, then quick release any remaining pressure.

7. Unlock and remove the lid. In a bowl, whisk together the cornstarch and remaining ¼ cup of water.

8. Select Sauté. Once the liquid is simmering, stir in the cornstarch mixture, and simmer for about 1 minute, or until the sauce has thickened. Press Cancel to stop cooking. Season with salt and pepper.

♻ **Ingredient Tip:** Pork tenderloin is a long, narrow boneless cut of meat and is not the same as a pork loin. They cannot be used interchangeably since they do not cook the same way.

Per Serving: Calories: 488; Carbohydrates: 16g; Fat: 21g; Fiber: 0g; Protein: 57g; Sugar: 12g; Sodium: 594mg

Sweet Potato, Sausage, and Kale Soup

Serves 6 to 8

Prep time: 20 minutes / **Pressure cook:** 17 minutes on Sauté; 8 minutes on High

Pressure release: Natural for 10 minutes, then Quick / **Total time:** 1 hour

 WORTH THE WAIT   ONE-POT MEAL

Sweet potatoes and kale come together with the help of flavorful sausage to make a wholesome, meal-in-a-bowl soup. Kielbasa works great, but any hard sausage of a similar style, including Spanish chorizo, will work.

---

2 tablespoons extra-virgin olive oil

1 (10-ounce) fully cooked kielbasa or Spanish chorizo, cut into ¼-inch-thick slices

1 large yellow onion, chopped

3 garlic cloves, minced

2 pounds sweet potatoes, peeled and cut into 1-inch dice

1 pound Yukon Gold or white potatoes (not russets), peeled and cut into 1-inch dice

6 cups Chicken Stock (page 137) or store-bought low-sodium chicken stock

Kosher salt

Freshly ground black pepper

1 small bunch kale, stemmed and coarsely chopped

1. Preheat the Instant Pot by selecting Sauté. Line a plate with paper towels.

2. Once hot, pour in the oil, then add the sausage. Cook, stirring, for about 7 minutes, or until browned. Using a slotted spoon, transfer to the prepared plate to drain.

3. Add the onion and garlic to the pot. Cook for 5 minutes, or until the onion is translucent.

4. Add the sweet potatoes, potatoes, and stock. Season with salt and pepper.

5. Lock the lid into place. Select Pressure Cook or Manual, and cook at High Pressure for 8 minutes.

6. After cooking, naturally release the pressure for 10 minutes, then quick release any remaining pressure.

7. Unlock and remove the lid. Using a potato masher or immersion blender, mash about half of the potatoes, leaving some chunks.

8. Select Sauté, and add the kale. Cook for 5 minutes, or until the kale has wilted. Press Cancel to stop cooking.

9. Add the sausage, and serve.

Per Serving: Calories: 327; Fat: 11g; Protein: 16g; Carbohydrates: 43g; Fiber: 6.5g; Sugar: 7.5g; Sodium: 580mg

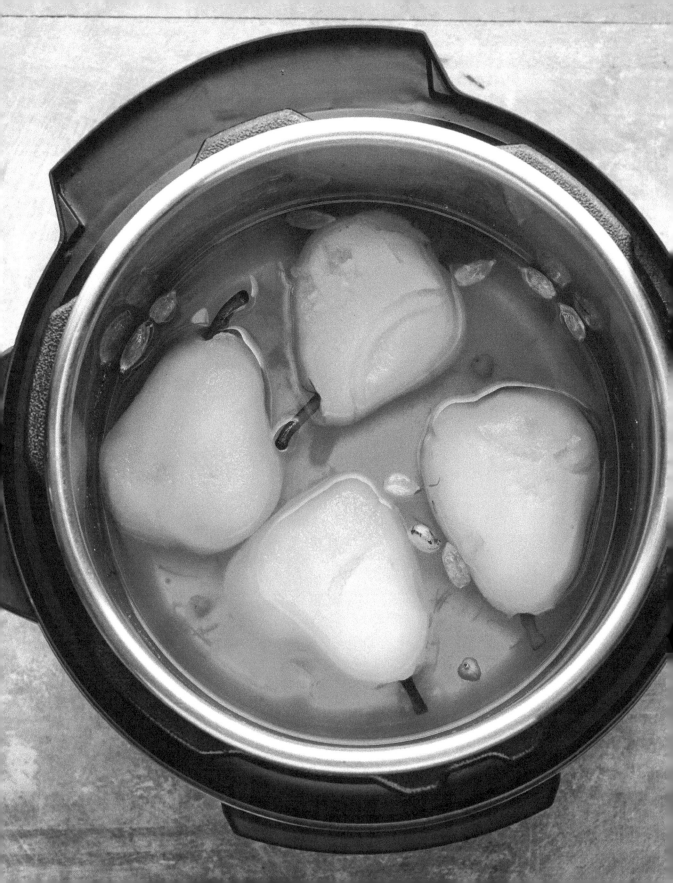

CHAPTER EIGHT

Desserts and Staples

POACHED PEARS WITH CARDAMOM

Serves 4

Prep time: 10 minutes / **Pressure cook:** 8 minutes on High; 15 to 20 minutes on Sauté
Pressure release: Quick / **Total time:** 45 minutes

 QUICK

Poached pears are one of my favorite fruit-based desserts. My version uses dry white wine and cardamom, which adds spicy, herbal, fragrant notes to the dish. If you do not have cardamom, try a 1-inch knob of peeled ginger and a cinnamon stick instead. Red wine may also be used in place of the white if preferred.

---

4 firm pears, peeled
2 cups water
1½ cups dry white wine
½ cup sugar
2 tablespoons freshly squeezed lemon juice

10 cardamom pods, lightly crushed, or
   1 teaspoon ground cardamom
⅛ teaspoon kosher salt
½ cup roasted unsalted pistachios, chopped

1. Using a melon baller or spoon, scoop out the seeds and core from the bottom of each pear.

2. In the Instant Pot, combine the water, wine, sugar, lemon juice, cardamom, and salt. Mix well. Press Sauté, and bring to a simmer.

3. Add the pears.

4. Lock the lid into place. Select Pressure Cook or Manual, and cook at High Pressure for 8 minutes.

5. After cooking, quick release the pressure.

6. Unlock and remove the lid. Transfer the pears to serving dishes.

7. Press Sauté, and bring the liquid to a boil. Reduce by about half, 15 to 20 minutes. Press Cancel to stop cooking.

8. Ladle the sauce over each pear, and garnish with the pistachios.

❖ **Variation Tip:** If you don't have pistachios, use any nuts or seeds you like. You can also top the pears with a dollop of yogurt or whipped cream in addition to or in place of the nuts.

Per Serving: Calories: 236; Fat: 7g; Protein: 4g; Carbohydrates: 42g; Fiber: 6g; Sugar: 35g; Sodium: 38mg

BROWNIES

Serves 6

Prep time: 10 minutes, plus at least 30 minutes to cool / **Pressure cook:** 35 minutes on High

Pressure release: Natural / **Total time:** 1 hour 25 minutes

 WORTH THE WAIT

These brownies are made with Greek yogurt—they taste decadent but are healthier for you. Remember, brownies cooked in the Instant Pot are more cake-like than ones baked in a conventional oven. But the chocolatey goodness is just as satisfying.

---

1 cup all-purpose flour
¾ cup confectioners' sugar
¼ cup cocoa powder
1 teaspoon baking powder
½ teaspoon baking soda

½ cup low-fat milk
¼ cup 2 percent plain Greek yogurt
3 tablespoons canola oil, plus 1 teaspoon
2 cups water
½ teaspoon coarse or flaky sea salt

1. In a large bowl, sift together the flour, sugar, and cocoa powder.

2. Add the baking powder and baking soda. Mix to combine.

3. In a medium bowl, whisk together the milk, yogurt, and 3 tablespoons of oil.

4. Add the wet ingredients to the dry ingredients in three additions, gently folding them together with each addition to form a smooth batter.

5. Grease a 7-inch springform pan with the remaining 1 teaspoon of oil.

6. Pour the batter into the pan, and tightly cover with aluminum foil.

7. Pour the water into the inner pot, and place the trivet inside. Place the pan on the trivet.

8. Lock the lid into place. Select Pressure Cook or Manual, and cook at High Pressure for 35 minutes.

9. After cooking, naturally release the pressure.

10. Unlock and remove the lid. Remove the pan and foil. Sprinkle the brownies with the sea salt, and let cool for at least 30 minutes. Gently remove from the pan, slice, and serve.

🌿 **Flavor Boost:** Coffee can add depth to any chocolate recipe; for this brownie recipe, add 1 to 1½ teaspoons instant coffee granules along with the dry ingredients. Cook time and pressure remain the same.

Per Serving: Calories: 225; Fat: 8.5g; Protein: 5g; Carbohydrates: 34g; Fiber: 2g; Sugar: 16g; Sodium: 211mg

PEACH AND BLACKBERRY CRISP

Serves 4

Prep time: 5 minutes / **Pressure cook:** 10 minutes on High

Pressure release: Natural for 5 minutes, then Quick / **Total time:** 30 minutes

 QUICK

Who can say no to warm peaches and blackberries with a crumble oat topping? Although this dessert calls for fresh fruit, frozen can be substituted in a pinch.

1½ cups water
¼ cup all-purpose flour
¼ cup rolled oats
¼ cup brown sugar
3 tablespoons unsalted butter, cut into small pieces
½ teaspoon ground cinnamon

3 medium peaches, peeled, pitted, and cut into ½-inch-thick slices
1 cup blackberries
2 tablespoons maple syrup
1 teaspoon freshly squeezed lemon juice
Nonstick cooking spray, for coating the cake pan

1. Prepare the Instant Pot by pouring the water into the pot and placing the steam rack on top.

2. In a medium bowl, using a fork or pastry blender, combine the flour, oats, sugar, butter, and cinnamon until crumbly.

3. In a medium bowl, combine the peaches, blackberries, maple syrup, and lemon juice.

4. Grease a 7-inch cake pan with cooking spray.

5. Pour the fruit mixture into the prepared pan. Top evenly with the crumble mixture.

6. Cover the pan tightly with aluminum foil. Place on the steam rack.

7. Lock the lid into place. Select Pressure Cook or Manual, and cook at High Pressure for 10 minutes.

8. After cooking, naturally release the pressure for 5 minutes, then quick release any remaining pressure.

9. Unlock and remove the lid. Carefully remove the cake pan and foil. Let cool slightly before serving.

❖ **Variation Tip:** Place the pan under an oven broiler for 3 minutes for a crispy topping.

Per Serving: Calories: 287; Fat: 13g; Protein: 3g; Carbohydrates: 44g; Fiber: 4g; Sugar: 30g; Sodium: 7mg

Cinnamon Yogurt Custard

Serves 4

Prep time: 10 minutes, plus 4 hours to cool and chill / **Pressure cook:** 25 minutes on High

Pressure release: Natural / **Total time:** 4 hours 45 minutes

5 OR FEWER INGREDIENTS   WORTH THE WAIT

Sometimes all you need are some simple ingredients to create a delicious and decadent dessert. This custard is the perfect example. With just a few ingredients and the fresh fruit of your choice, this recipe is sure to become a favorite. What's more, it's also perfect to make ahead for parties and potlucks.

½ cup 2 percent plain Greek yogurt
½ cup sweetened condensed milk
½ teaspoon ground cinnamon

2 cups water
¼ cup chopped fruit or berries of your choice

1. In a heatproof bowl that fits inside the Instant Pot, mix together the yogurt, condensed milk, and cinnamon. Tightly cover the bowl with aluminum foil.

2. Pour the water into the inner pot, and place a trivet inside. Place the bowl on the trivet.

3. Lock the lid into place. Select Pressure Cook or Manual, and cook at High Pressure for 25 minutes.

4. Unlock and remove the lid. Carefully remove the bowl. Let cool at room temperature for 30 minutes, then cover and refrigerate for 3 to 4 hours.

5. Serve the custard garnished with the fruit of your choice.

❧ **Ingredient Tip:** You can also include ¼ to ½ cup sweet fresh fruit puree, such as mango, blueberry, or even banana. Citrus fruits won't work well because the acid will cause the dairy to curdle. If you use a fresh fruit puree, increase the cook time to 30 minutes.

Per Serving: Calories: 149; Fat: 4g; Protein: 6g; Carbohydrates: 23g; Fiber: 0g; Sugar: 22g; Sodium: 59mg

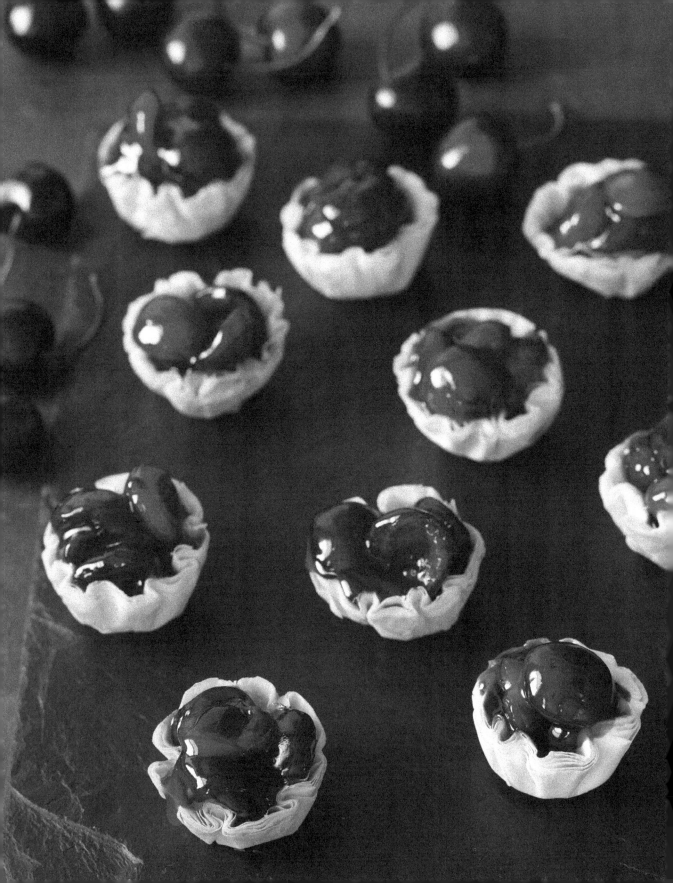

Brandy-Soaked Cheater Cherry Pies

Serves 8

Prep time: 35 minutes / **Pressure cook:** 15 minutes on Sauté Low
Pressure release: None / **Total time:** 50 minutes

WORTH THE WAIT

Cherry pie is a classic pie filling, but making pie crust can be a lot of work and hard to execute. It also uses a lot of butter. The good news is that the cherry filling is the easy part! By combining it with phyllo shells from the freezer section of any grocery store, most of the work is already done!

2 pounds cherries, pitted
1/3 cup brandy
2/3 cup sugar
3 tablespoons cornstarch

Juice of ½ lime
Pinch kosher salt
2 (2-ounce) boxes mini phyllo shells

1. In a large bowl, combine the cherries and brandy. Let soak, stirring occasionally, for 30 minutes.

2. Preheat the Instant Pot by selecting Sauté, and adjust to Less for low heat.

3. Pour the cherries and the liquid at the bottom of the bowl into the inner pot.

4. Stir in the sugar, cornstarch, lime juice, and salt. Cook, stirring frequently, for 10 to 15 minutes, or until thickened. Press Cancel to stop cooking.

5. Let the filling cool for a few minutes before spooning into the phyllo shells.

♻ **Ingredient Tip:** Frozen cherries are fine to use; thaw them completely before soaking.

Per Serving: Calories: 228; Fat: 2.5g; Protein: 2g; Carbohydrates: 44g; Fiber: 2g; Sugar: 30g; Sodium: 63mg

APPLESAUCE

Serves 8

Prep time: 5 minutes / **Pressure cook:** 8 minutes on High

Pressure release: Natural for 10 minutes, then Quick / **Total time:** 30 minutes

 5 OR FEWER INGREDIENTS   QUICK

Making homemade applesauce is as easy as throwing some apple chunks into your Instant Pot with a little water and setting the timer! This recipe is perfectly delicious eaten alone or used as a substitute for oil in baked goods. Since it is naturally sweetened, it makes for a healthy snack for kids, too.

---

3 pounds apples, peeled, cored, and quartered

½ cup water

½ teaspoon ground cinnamon (optional)

¼ teaspoon ground nutmeg (optional)

1. Put the apples, water, cinnamon (if using), and nutmeg (if using) in the inner pot.

2. Lock the lid into place. Select Pressure Cook or Manual, and cook at High Pressure for 8 minutes.

3. After cooking, naturally release the pressure for 10 minutes, then quick release any remaining pressure.

4. Unlock and remove the lid. Using an immersion blender, traditional blender, or food processor, blend the apple mixture until smooth. Serve immediately, refrigerate in a sealed container for up to 5 days, or freeze for up to 3 months.

❖ **Ingredient Tip:** I like to use Fuji apples, but it's tasty with other apples such as Gala, Honeycrisp, Granny Smith, or a combination. If your apples are on the tart side, you can sweeten the applesauce with a little maple syrup after cooking.

Per Serving: Calories: 80; Fat: 0g; Protein: 0g; Carbohydrates: 21g; Fiber: 3.5g; Sugar: 16g; Sodium: 2mg

Hot Sauce

Makes about 20 ounces

Prep time: 5 minutes / **Pressure cook:** 2 minutes on Sauté; 1 minute on High

Pressure release: Natural / **Total time:** 20 minutes

 5 OR FEWER INGREDIENTS   QUICK

Calling all hot sauce lovers! With this easy homemade hot sauce, you may never have to buy the condiment again. The best part is you can make it truly unique and customize with any pepper or combination of peppers, depending on how spicy you want your hot sauce to be.

---

1 tablespoon extra-virgin olive oil

1 small yellow onion, diced

6 garlic cloves, minced

1 medium carrot, chopped

8 ounces hot peppers, chopped and stemmed

1 cup apple cider vinegar, plus more as needed

Kosher salt

1. Select Sauté, and pour the oil into the inner pot.

2. Once the oil is hot, add the onion and garlic. Sauté for 2 minutes.

3. Add the carrot, peppers, and vinegar.

4. Lock the lid into place. Select Pressure Cook or Manual, and cook at High Pressure for 1 minute.

5. After cooking, naturally release the pressure.

6. Unlock and remove the lid. Using an immersion or regular blender, puree the mixture until smooth.

7. Add more vinegar to thin out the sauce if needed. Season with salt.

8. Pour the hot sauce in sterile glass jars or bottles, and store in the refrigerator for up to 6 months.

❖ **Ingredient Tip:** The peppers you choose will help determine how hot your hot sauce will be. Mild hot peppers—such as poblano and Anaheim—will give you a flavorful, mild hot sauce. Medium hot peppers—such as serrano and jalapeño—will add a bit more heat. Extra-hot peppers—such as Thai and habanero—should be used with caution.

Per Serving (1 tablespoon): Calories: 8; Fat: 0.5g; Protein: 0g; Carbohydrates: 1g; Fiber: 0g; Sugar: 0.5g; Sodium: 86mg

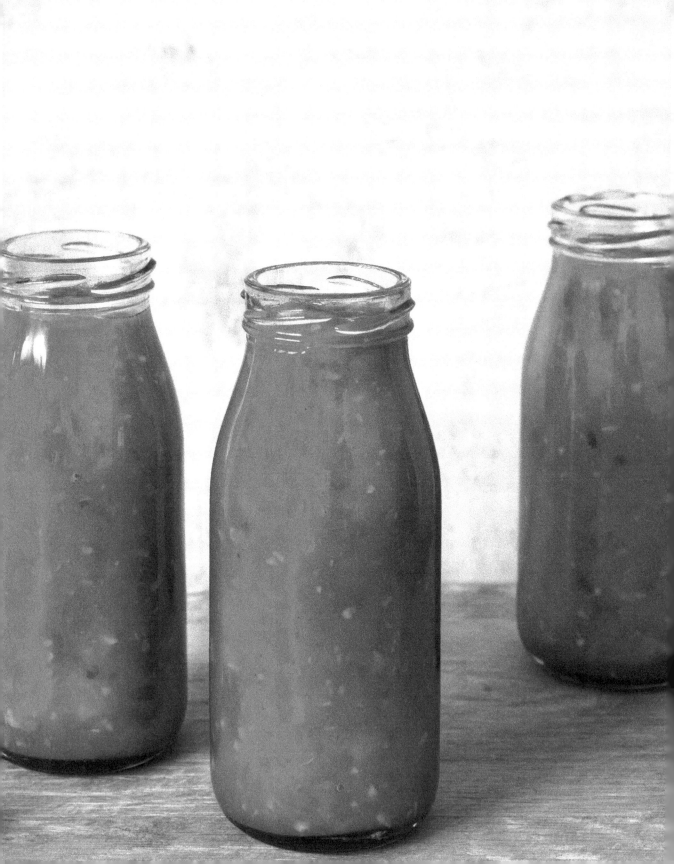

Classic Marinara Sauce

Makes about 4 cups

Prep time: 10 minutes / **Pressure cook:** 3 minutes on Sauté; 30 minutes on High

Pressure release: Natural for 10 minutes, then Quick / **Total time:** 1 hour

 5 OR FEWER INGREDIENTS   WORTH THE WAIT

Marinara is in a huge number of Italian and Italian-inspired dishes, so it pays to have a good recipe handy. Most traditional recipes call for an hour or more of simmering on the stove, but this sauce only cooks for 30 minutes. Use it on pasta, pizza, and more.

---

2 tablespoons extra-virgin olive oil

1 medium yellow onion, grated

1 large carrot, peeled and grated

5 garlic cloves, grated

1 (28-ounce) can crushed tomatoes

½ teaspoon dried oregano

Pinch sugar (optional)

Kosher salt

Freshly ground black pepper

1. Preheat the Instant Pot by selecting Sauté.

2. Once hot, pour in the oil, then add the onion and carrot. Sauté for 2 minutes, or until the onion is translucent.

3. Add the garlic, and cook for 30 seconds.

4. Add the tomatoes and oregano. Mix well.

5. Lock the lid into place. Select Pressure Cook or Manual, and cook at High Pressure for 30 minutes.

6. After cooking, naturally release the pressure for 10 minutes, then quick release any remaining pressure.

7. Unlock and remove the lid. Stir, and taste for seasoning. Add the sugar (if using). Season with salt and pepper. Refrigerate in a sealed container for up to a week, or freeze for up to 3 months.

❖ **Flavor Boost:** Add a pinch of red pepper flakes for a little heat or a sprinkle of basil for freshness.

Per Serving (½ cup): Calories: 78; Fat: 35g; Protein: 2g; Carbohydrates: 10g; Fiber: 3g; Sugar: 5g; Sodium: 254mg

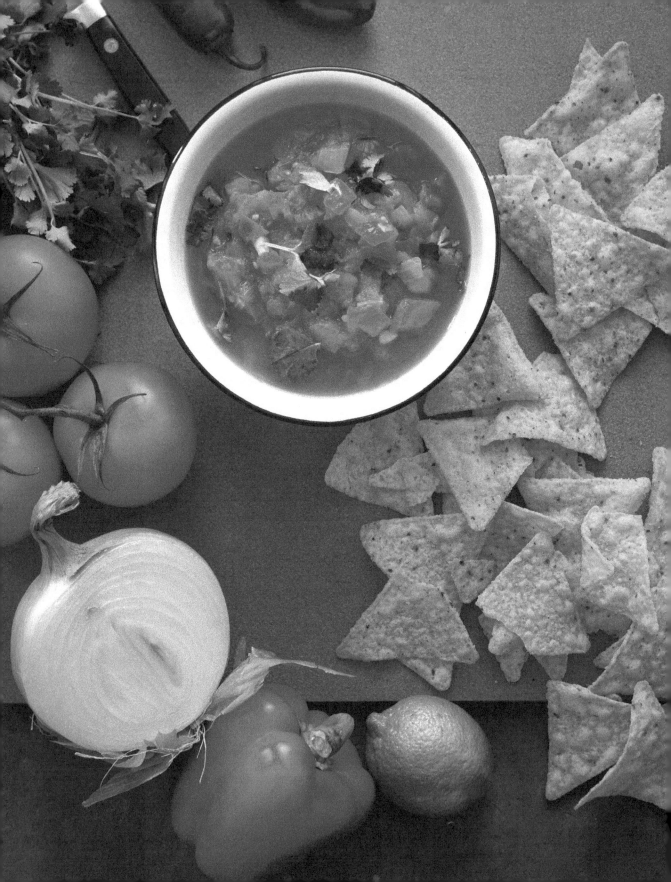

Garden Salsa

Serves 6 to 8

Prep time: 15 minutes / **Pressure cook:** 5 minutes on High

Pressure release: Natural for 10 minutes, then Quick / **Total time:** 40 minutes

 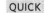 QUICK

The salsa aisle at the grocery store can be a bit overwhelming. So many brands and flavors to choose from, and how do you know what heat level is right for you? The best solution is to make your own. It guarantees your salsa will be delicious and fresh, and you have full control over the heat. This version is fairly mild, so feel free to add hotter chile peppers or chili powder.

8 large tomatoes, coarsely chopped

5 or 6 garlic cloves, finely diced

2 jalapeño peppers, seeded and diced

1 bell pepper, any color, cored and diced

1 small red onion, diced

1 small yellow onion, diced

1 tablespoon ground cumin

¼ cup tomato paste

¼ cup chopped fresh cilantro

2 tablespoons freshly squeezed lime juice

Kosher salt

Freshly ground black pepper

1. In the Instant Pot, stir together the tomatoes, garlic, jalapeños, bell pepper, red onion, yellow onion, and cumin.

2. Lock the lid into place. Select Pressure Cook or Manual, and cook at High Pressure for 5 minutes.

3. After cooking, naturally release the pressure for 10 minutes, then quick release any remaining pressure.

4. Carefully remove the lid. Stir in the tomato paste, cilantro, and lime juice. Season with salt and pepper. Let cool completely before serving.

❖ **Ingredient Tip:** Use a food processor to speed up all the veggie chopping.

Per Serving: Calories: 64; Fat: 0.5g; Protein: 3g; Carbohydrates: 14g; Fiber: 3.5g; Sugar: 7g; Sodium: 61mg

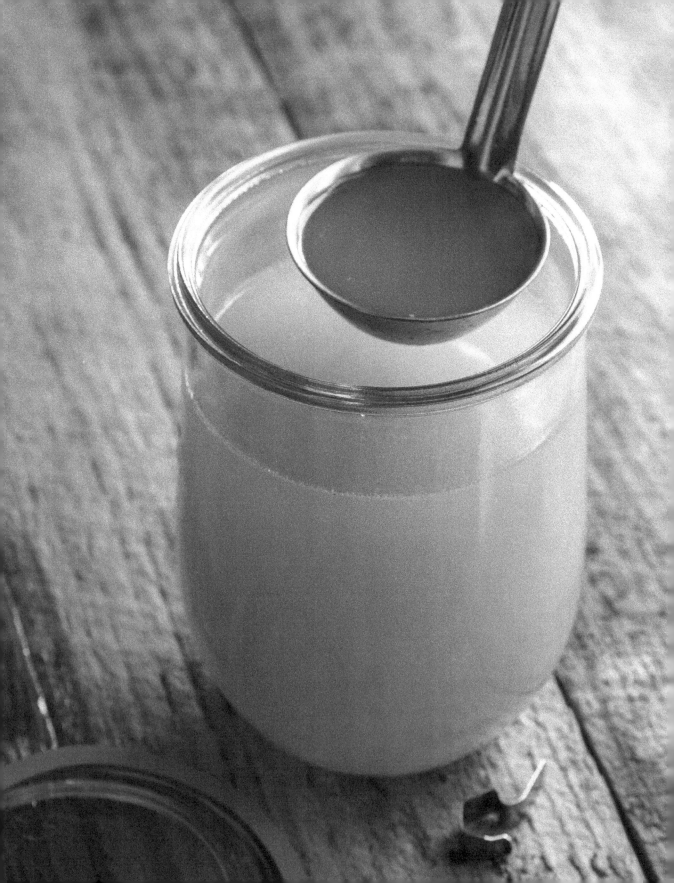

CHICKEN STOCK

Makes 1 quart

Prep time: 20 minutes / **Pressure cook:** 1 hour 30 minutes on High

Pressure release: Natural for 15 minutes, then Quick

Total time: 2 hours 15 minutes, plus overnight to chill

 5 OR FEWER INGREDIENTS   WORTH THE WAIT

If you haven't used your Instant Pot to make stock, you don't know what you're missing. Ninety minutes and very little work yield a savory stock that tastes like it simmered for hours. Many recipes for chicken stock call for the addition of vegetables and herbs, but this version keeps to the bare bones (pun intended). Feel free to include the extra ingredients if you prefer.

---

2 pounds meaty chicken bones (backs, wing tips, leg quarters)

¼ to ¾ teaspoon kosher salt
1 quart water, or more if needed

1. Pile the chicken bones in the Instant Pot. Sprinkle with ¼ teaspoon of salt.

2. Add the water, just to cover the bones but not filling the pot more than half full of water. Use more if necessary.

3. Lock the lid into place. Select Pressure Cook or Manual, and cook at High Pressure for 1 hour 30 minutes.

4. After cooking, naturally release the pressure for 15 minutes, then quick release any remaining pressure.

5. Unlock and remove the lid. Line a colander with cheesecloth, and place over a large bowl.

6. Pour the chicken parts and stock into the colander. Discard the solids.

7. Let the stock cool and then refrigerate for several hours or overnight so that the fat hardens on the top of the stock.

8. Remove the layer of fat and discard.

9. If you like, add the remaining ½ teaspoon of salt to approximate the salt level of commercial low-sodium stocks. The stock can be refrigerated for several days or frozen for several months in airtight containers.

Per Serving (1 cup): Calories: 30; Fat: 0g; Protein: 6g; Carbohydrates: 1g; Fiber: 0g; Sugar: 0g; Sodium: 140mg

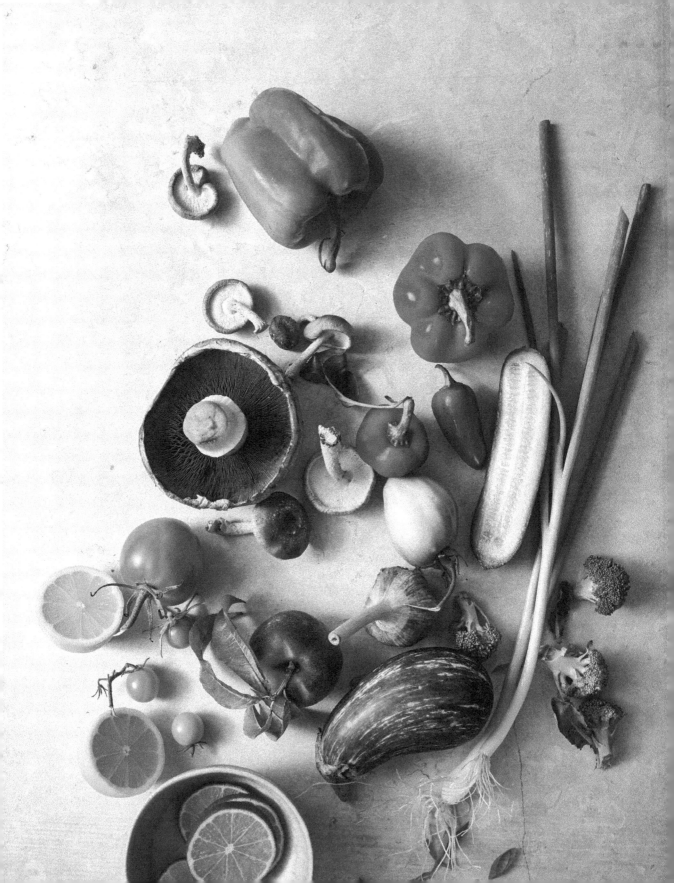

MEASUREMENT CONVERSIONS

VOLUME EQUIVALENTS (LIQUID)

US STANDARD	US STANDARD (OUNCES)	METRIC (APPROXIMATE)
2 tablespoons	1 fl. oz.	30 mL
¼ cup	2 fl. oz.	60 mL
½ cup	4 fl. oz.	120 mL
1 cup	8 fl. oz.	240 mL
1½ cups	12 fl. oz.	355 mL
2 cups or 1 pint	16 fl. oz.	475 mL
4 cups or 1 quart	32 fl. oz.	1 L
1 gallon	128 fl. oz.	4 L

VOLUME EQUIVALENTS (DRY)

US STANDARD	METRIC (APPROXIMATE)
⅛ teaspoon	0.5 mL
¼ teaspoon	1 mL
½ teaspoon	2 mL
¾ teaspoon	4 mL
1 teaspoon	5 mL
1 tablespoon	15 mL
¼ cup	59 mL
⅓ cup	79 mL
½ cup	118 mL
⅔ cup	156 mL
¾ cup	177 mL
1 cup	235 mL
2 cups or 1 pint	475 mL
3 cups	700 mL
4 cups or 1 quart	1 L

OVEN TEMPERATURES

FAHRENHEIT (F)	CELSIUS (C) (APPROXIMATE)
250°F	120°C
300°F	150°C
325°F	165°C
350°F	180°C
375°F	190°C
400°F	200°C
425°F	220°C
450°F	230°C

WEIGHT EQUIVALENTS

US STANDARD	METRIC (APPROXIMATE)
½ ounce	15 g
1 ounce	30 g
2 ounces	60 g
4 ounces	115 g
8 ounces	225 g
12 ounces	340 g
16 ounces or 1 pound	455 g

RESOURCES

Cooking healthy meals has never been easier. Here you'll find helpful information to make the most out of your Instant Pot.

The official Instant Pot website features a cooking time chart, videos, FAQs for different models, and a recipe database: InstantPot.com

Conner, Polly, and Rachel Tiemeyer. *From Freezer to Cooker: Delicious Whole-Foods Meals for the Slow Cooker, Pressure Cooker, and Instant Pot.* New York: Rodale Books, 2020.

Eisner, Jeffrey. *The Lighter Step-By-Step Instant Pot Cookbook: Easy Recipes for a Slimmer, Healthier You—With Photographs of Every Step.* New York: Voracious, 2021.

There are many Facebook groups with enthusiastic Instant Pot users willing to share their tips, recipes, and ideas. Here are a few I recommend:

- Instant Pot Weight Watchers Recipes
- Instant Pot Healthy Recipes
- All Things Instant Pot

INDEX

Acknowledgments

This book is the result of the efforts of many people. Thank you to my editor, Kelly Koester, for her guidance and support, and to the entire publishing team at Rockridge Press for their hard work in making this cookbook come to life.

Thanks to my family and friends, for sharing with me the love of food and for your continuing support of all my kitchen endeavors over the years. I can't wait to cook for you again.

Finally, a special mention to my husband, James, for being the best recipe taster I could ask for. Thank you for always encouraging me in everything I do.

About the Author

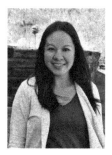

Karen Lee Young is the founder of *The Tasty Bite*, a food blog featuring recipes that make cooking from scratch as simple as possible for both novice and experienced home cooks. Her work has been featured on *Huffington Post*, *Country Living*, *Buzzfeed*, *Greatist*, and many other media outlets. Originally from New York City, she now lives in Colorado with her husband and daughter. When Karen is not in the kitchen, you'll find her enjoying the outdoors, exploring different restaurants, and traveling near and far.

CPSIA information can be obtained
at www.ICGtesting.com
Printed in the USA
LVHW021614150921
697888LV00002B/2